Choose the Change: Cookbook
&
Weight Loss Guide

ASHLEY DONAHOO

ISBN-13: 978-1494857707
ISBN-10: 1494857707

You can follow Ashley on social media!

Official Website: www.ChooseTheChange.net
Facebook: www.facebook.com/ChooseTheChange
Instagram: ADonahoo_CTC
Twitter: @Donahoo_CTC
Tumblr Blog: AshleyDonahoo.tumblr.com

DISCLAIMER

Before embarking on any weight loss regimen or program, consult your personal physician. Ashley Donahoo is not nor claims to be a licensed physician, psychiatrist/ psychologist, nutritionist, or personal trainer. The information provided in this book is designed to provide helpful information on healthy recipes and weight loss. This book is not meant to be used, nor should it be used, to diagnose or treat any medical condition. For diagnosis or treatment of any medical problem, consult your own physician. The publisher and author are not responsible for any specific health or allergy needs that may require medical supervision and are not liable for any damages or negative consequences from any treatment, action, application or preparation, to any person reading or following the information in this book. The use of the recipes included in this book are done at one's own risk and assessment of dietary requirements. Consuming raw or undercooked meats are not recommended, and pose the possibility of serious illness or even death. Ensuring the proper cooking of all recipes included in this book are the responsibility of each individual reader/ cook. References are provided for informational purposes only and do not constitute endorsement of any websites or other sources. Readers should be aware that the websites listed in this book may change. The rest of this is just legal jargon you will not need. This is a test of your persistence. You're still reading this? This book is not to be used as a floating device. Do not attempt to use this book to put out a fire, especially a kitchen fire. You're going to do great, just stick with it like you did in reading this Disclaimer.

ASHLEY DONAHOO

DEDICATION

I dedicate this book to my family and friends who have loved, supported, and helped me along every journey I've ever embarked upon. I could not have accomplished all the things I have in life without the blessings I call my family and friends.

I also dedicate this book to all the people who feel as though they have no hope of changing their lives. I pray my story and the information in this book shows you that you can CHOOSE THE CHANGE in your life and health, take back control, and find happiness and love for yourself.

CONTENTS

ACKNOWLEDGMENTS

This book would not have been possible without the help and support of my amazing family and friends. Specifically, to my husband, David, who has stood by me through thick and thin (literally and figuratively), loved me for who I was regardless of my pants size or mental/ emotional state, and has always supported me (even if that means doing the laundry and dishes) through any and all of my dreams and ventures, never wanting recognition or thanks: Thank you, baby. Thank you for holding me and wiping away my tears when I needed sheltering and comfort, pushing me when I needed motivation, cheering for me when I succeeded, and loving me when I know I was unlovable to the rest of the world.

To my sons, Zachary and Connor, whom I live and breathe for: In my darkest times, your smiles and love gave me reason for living. Boys, knowing that I will now be around longer to watch you continue to grow, become men, have lives and families of your own, experience all the joy life brings, and fulfill your great purposes in life has always been one of my greatest motivators. Thank you for being such amazing young men and my greatest blessings in life.

To my amazing parents, Dean and Karen, my greatest cheerleaders: Your love and support has been the rock on which any of my accomplishments have ever been founded. I proudly say I'm a great mix of you both, and I strive to encompass both of your greatest qualities. Ever since I was a child, all I've ever wanted was for you to be proud of me. Through all of life's ups and downs, I know your love and desire for me to succeed in every arena of life never waivers. Thank you for being the best parents I could've ever asked for.

To my Aunt Karmela, who helped guide and support me through my weight loss journey (and other areas of life): Your gentle guidance and loving support was vital at times through this journey, and in the moments when there was no one else that could've helped me pick myself back up and find an answer to keep going, you did. Thank you for allowing me to find my own way, but always being there when I had nowhere else to turn and believing in my ability to conquer this when others didn't.

To all of my friends and family who encouraged me along the way, cheered me on, gave me tips and help, loved on me, and remained constant even through all my changes: "Thank you" just isn't enough. The support I had on this journey was by far one of the biggest keys to my success, and I'll be forever grateful. The highs and lows of friendships can be challenging at times, but you're the family I can and always will choose to have in my life. I love and appreciate you all.

I want to specifically thank the people who had a direct hand in the completion of this book through their help and support:

Melissa Bartush: Test Cooker
Karen Dampier: Test Cooker, Photographer
David Donahoo: Test Cooker, Photographer
Tiffany Morgan: Test Cooker
Janene Putman: Test Cooker, Consultant in Publishing
Andersen Roberts: Test Cooker
Karmela Rotter: Test Cooker
Daniel Wright: Graphic Designer

1. INTRODUCTION

My name is Ashley Donahoo, and I lost 137 lbs, over 100", and went down 11 sizes through proper nutrition and exercise alone, with no help from programs, pills, surgery, doctors, personal trainers, nutritionists, or even a gym membership. I started with a free online tracking tool, a couple borrowed workout DVDs, and a pair of tennis shoes. It really is true: If I can do it, ANYONE can.

My hope in this book is to provide you with the tools and knowledge I learned, used, and developed along my journey that helped me lose my weight and take control of my life and health so that YOU can do the same thing! This book includes over 80 recipes, and all complete meals (sides included) are under 500 calories (most are much less). All recipes include a nutrition label for information as well as ease of tracking (which I strongly recommend). I have also included nutritional information and explanations, explained how your body works with the food you give it (and should be giving it), sample menus and a grocery list, and much more. I share my story and these tips and information in an effort to show people that it really is all about making it a lifestyle change, not a "diet."

Through this journey, your views on food, your self-worth, and life will change for the better. This is much more an emotional and mental journey a than a physical one. You CAN lose weight and take control of your life and health if you simply CHOOSE to. So CHOOSE THE CHANGE for yourself!

2. ASHLEY'S STORY

In the Spring of 2010, at the age of 25, I was a completely different person than I am now. I was morbidly obese at almost 300 lbs, and was diagnosed with and being treated for Major Depression, Polycystic Ovarian Syndrome, Chronic Migraines, Liver Disease, High Blood Pressure, Anemia, and was Pre-Diabetic. I was also on prescription medicine for all those health problems. I felt completely lost and utterly hopeless about how to change my weight and health as a whole, and blamed everything but myself and my choices. I had allowed myself to BELIEVE I was just a victim of poor health, bad genetics, uncontrollable stress, low income, a too-packed schedule, unfortunate circumstances, and a plethora of other things I used as excuses for why I couldn't lose weight. My doctor finally threw his hands up at me in exasperation. "Ashley, I cannot prescribe you any more medicine. The only thing that is going to help you is to lose weight. You've got to get this under control, or I don't think you'll live to see 30," he finally said to me. No amount of medicine was truly helping me anymore. I had gotten to where I was from MY choices. I was slowly committing suicide.

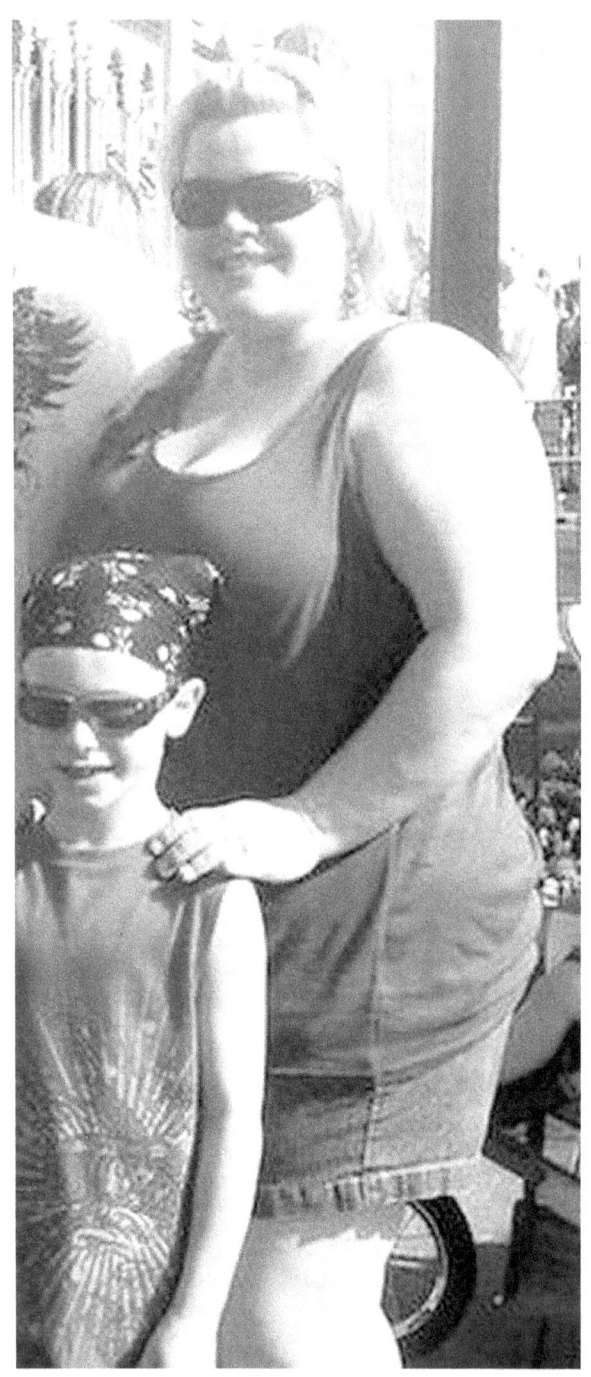

April 2010: Almost 300 lbs

I was in such a dark place, even my doctor's grave warning gave me no pause. I quickly shook it off as I got in my car and thought, "He's a doctor. Of course he's going to say I need to lose weight. Easy for him to say – he's skinny!" and I'm sure I went through a drive-thru on the way home. I was angry. Angry that my life wasn't going the way I had planned or thought it would. Angry that we weren't even making it paycheck to paycheck. Angry at my job, my family, my friends. Why? I'm sure I didn't even have logical reasons. I was just – angry at life. So angry, in fact, that I hated those who seemed happy. I was jealous of others' accomplishments and joy in their lives, but I was too lost, everything was too dark in my life so I thought, that I barely functioned in the fake happiness I tried to convey to the rest of the world. This act wasn't very convincing to most people, as my unhappiness eventually came out in complaints, anger, or withdrawal in one way or another.

I eventually had to take FMLA from work for a while to balance out my depression medications, and had to be "watched" by my husband at times due to my suicidal thoughts. Looking back on those times is still hard. I felt out of control of everything in my life, but food was the one thing I could control. I controlled what I put in my mouth, and if it tasted and felt good, I was going to have it and no one would tell me otherwise. It felt naughty to sneak food, like a forbidden fruit. Deep down, I knew I shouldn't be eating those things in those quantities, but I wanted to do it. I was obsessed with food. I wanted to sneak and eat like a kid stealing a cookie from the cookie jar.

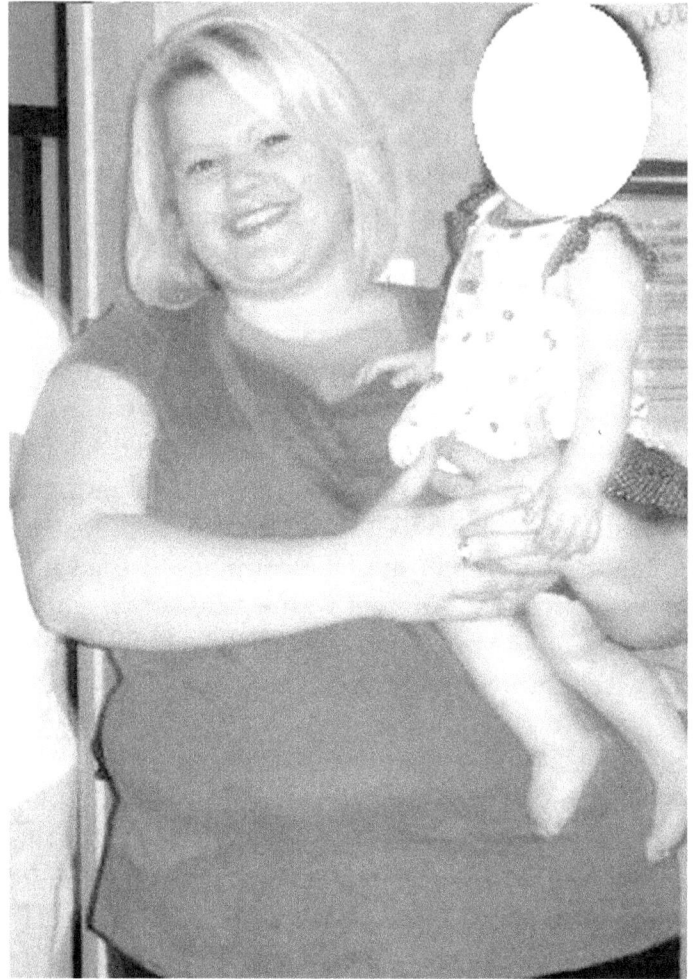

June 2010: Almost 300 lbs

Worried about my worsening health (mentally and physically), my husband talked me into going for a walk one day in early June 2010. Half way down our city block, although we were walking at a snail's pace, I was out of breath, and had severe pain shooting from my feet up to my legs and back. My head was thumping as my blood pressure spiked. I realized, in that moment, as I whined and complained to turn back, just how far I had let myself go.

In high school, I played soccer and softball, was in marching band, and was all around a very active and healthy teenager. I never struggled with being overweight until my later teen years because I was so active. Like most teen girls, I thought I was fat, though. I struggled with anorexia for a time, trying to be "skinny" and fit the mold society and media told me I should. Fear of being fat and ugly, and being made fun of and called fat and ugly by my peers (even though, looking back, I was at a healthy weight) fueled the fire of obsession with food that would eventually consume me and drive me toward my food addiction. After having a child and getting married very young, living in poverty, struggling in literally every facet of life, I eventually turned to food more and more to cope with my frustration and disappointment with myself and where my life had gone. I was so wrapped up in things not going the way I wanted and planned, that I couldn't see just how blessed I was in life. I was blinded to my own joy.

"How did I get HERE?!" I wondered, standing in the middle of the sidewalk that sunny June day. I was unhappy, and everything I was doing, even if it provided temporary fulfillment, was making it worse. I was doing this to myself. I couldn't hide behind my excuses anymore. I couldn't keep saying, "Well it's harder for me to lose weight because of my PCOS… My whole family struggles with weight, so I'm naturally going to be larger… I'm never going to be skinny, I'm not made to be… I can't afford a gym/ personal trainer/ surgery/ nutritionist/ program, so I can't lose weight… I'll never be on a weight loss reality show and get the help they are, so I can't lose weight like that…" and so on. I burst into tears from the realization hitting me in the head like a softball. This was my moment of awakening. I had to change something. I couldn't, and WOULDN'T, live like this anymore. By the time I got back home from that walk, my tears were dried, and I began to come up with a plan.

I had to find a way to lose weight that would work for me forever, not temporarily. I refused to be a yo-yo dieter like all the women I had watched growing up who struggled with their weight. I knew the fad diets (cabbage soup, anyone?), programs, and pills wouldn't work long term because I had tried them all, it seemed, and/or watched others do them, lose a few pounds, then gain it all back and then some when they went "back to normal." I refused to go down that road.

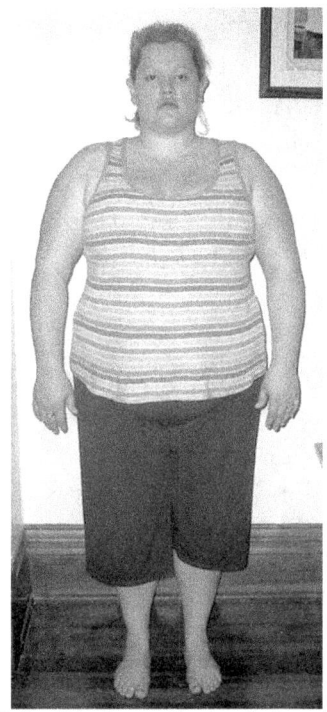

July 2010: 272 lbs (I had actually already lost about 16lbs here!)

My plan had to meet these guidelines: (1) It had to be free – my family couldn't afford a meal plan program, gym memberships, personal trainers, weight loss groups/ programs, "special"/ "diet" foods, workout equipment, etc. (2) It had to be easy and not time consuming– working full time, being married, and having two active kids didn't leave a lot of time in my day. (3) It had to be healthy – pills, surgery, and fad diets were out of the question for me because of the health risks and side effects (I was doing this to get healthy, not further my health issues, after all), but ALSO because they don't fit #4-->. (4) It had to be something I would do for the rest of my life (something I could maintain for life). I know I had to adopt a better lifestyle and healthy relationship with food and my body for this to last. I refuse(d) to be a yo-yo dieter. I knew I wouldn't stick to a particular "diet" for the rest of my life (as I had proven time and again already), and I knew I wouldn't work out every day for the rest of my life (much less hours a day). This had to be a new overall way of looking at food and treating my body – a total overhaul of my lifestyle, NOT A DIET just to lose a certain number of pounds. This would be to SAVE and CHANGE my life, not just to change my dress size. On June 12, 2010, I began to change my life one step, one choice at a time. I began to track everything that passed my lips and that I did for exercise on a FREE health and wellness website that has a seemingly endless database of nutrition and exercise information. I had officially RUN OUT OF EXCUSES.

I utilized this particular site and the entire internet to educate myself about good nutrition, BMR (Basal Metabolic Rate), nutrition labels, quality of food, exercise, etc. The supply of information is endless – there is no reason for anyone to be ignorant about it in this day and time with the amount of technology we all have at our fingertips. I started to change the way I looked at, cooked, and ate food. I made simple substitutions for higher calorie foods and ingredients for healthier ones. I started measuring and weighing my food so I could be absolutely sure that what I was tracking was accurate. This held me accountable for what I was eating instead of mindlessly shoveling it in whenever I felt the urge. Tracking also served as a food journal for me to refer back to if I had a tough week on the scale to assess where I could've gone wrong. I also started slowly exercising. I started walking and doing a (borrowed) 30 minute yoga DVD a few times a week. I quickly found myself actually enjoying it (something I never thought would happen) and, of course, the amazing results. Results not just found on the scale or in my clothes (which was fabulous), but also in my mind, my outlook on life, my attitude, my energy levels, how I felt physically – EVERYTHING about me was changing for the better, and I was starting to love and care about myself again. Every small thing I started doing in the beginning grew and grew into greater changes, challenges, and results. Each tiny step made the following step easier, and each success built me up and prepared me for the next challenge.

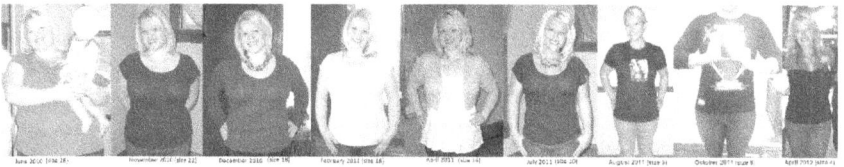

Progression in jeans' size from June 2010 (size 26 jeans) to April 2012 (size 4 jeans)

Along this journey, I realized I have an addiction to food. Notice I used present tense: "have." I will always have a tendency to turn to food for comfort, but through this journey, I learned self-control, modification, and moderation in my nutrition, but also a sense of self-worth that makes me WANT to make healthier choices for myself. Before I started my journey, not only did I not value myself enough to want to take care of my body, but I also had a serious lack of control when it came to unhealthy foods, overeating, and even sneaking food. I used it as comfort, but also as a way to have a sense of control. So many things in my life had been out of my control, but I was the boss of what I ate. I didn't realize this at the beginning, but, with time and self-reflection, it became more and more clear: The control I was exerting over my food in a negative way by overeating and sneaking food CHANGED into control over my food in a positive way through changing my lifestyle and relationship with food. I finally had REAL control over what was going in my mouth, and making conscious decisions and changes. Food became a fuel for my body to function on a higher level, a tool I used to better myself in every way, rather than a drug to tear my body apart.

This journey has not been easy, and there have been moments of weakness and times I "messed up." The beauty of THIS way of losing weight and changing your lifestyle is that it is OKAY to mess up! Each "mistake" is a learning opportunity and furthers your journey if you let it. This is my LIFE – not a certain plan or program I have to stick to word-for-word. I don't lose points or discount my entire day if I have dessert. If I don't get a workout in and/ or if I go over my calorie goal one day, then I track it, learn from it, and move on and make better choices the next day. There is NOTHING off limits in my new healthy lifestyle – I just have to be conscious of my choices, and use self control and moderation. So, no, losing weight and getting and staying healthy may not be "easy," but being obese, unhealthy, and unhappy isn't easy either – in fact, it's much harder to live the latter.

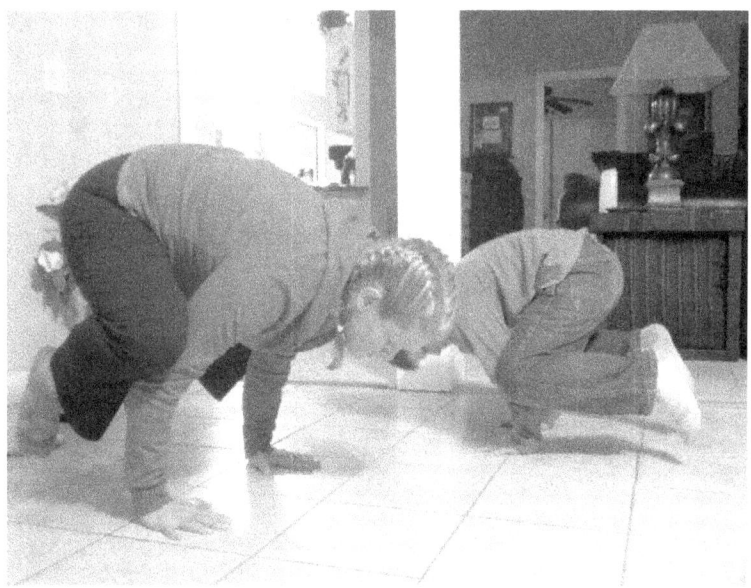

Moments from family activities. Me and my eldest having a contest on who can hold "The Frog" longer, which eventually got the whole family involved, falling on the floor, and laughing uncontrollably.

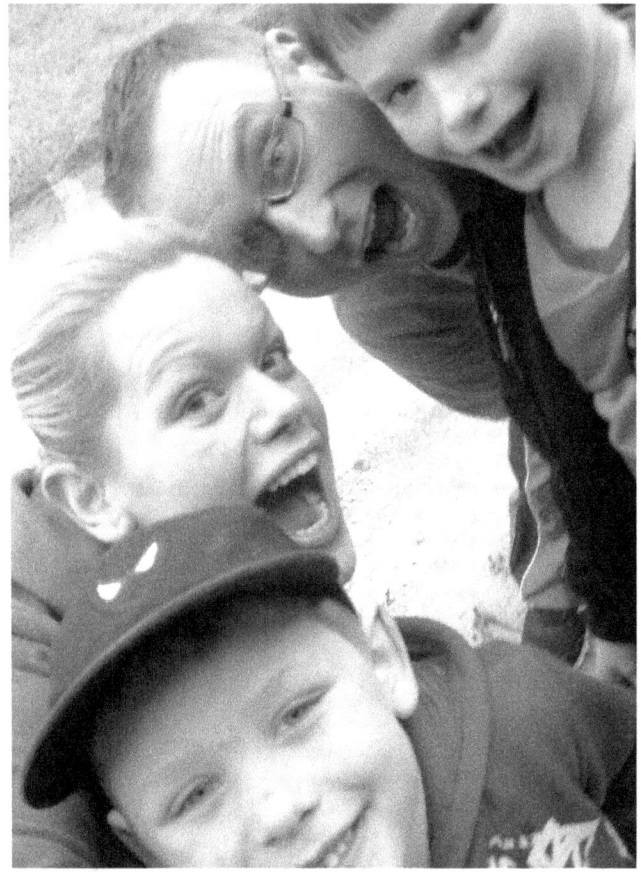

Moments from family activities. Our family out for a long walk instead of sitting on the couch.

The changes I have made in myself through this journey have had a ripple effect on my family and those around me. Funny how when you think you're just doing something that will affect you, it actually impacts everyone you come in contact with in some way. I now have a light that I can share with others instead of spending all my time trying to keep it from going out. My family life is so much happier and more fulfilling. I actually want to and can play with my children and take an active role in their childhood instead of sitting back and watching them grow up from the couch. We do fun activities together (i.e. walks, bowling, skating, hiking, playing ball, etc) as a family now instead of passive activities (i.e. movies, tv, video games). I'm a happier and more receptive mother and wife all around. My marriage has improved because I'm not so busy hating on myself and being self-conscious and angry about my body and life that I have more of myself to give to my husband and our relationship and family as a whole.

I'm a better friend, daughter, employee, and person than I ever was before taking control of my life. When I started loving and taking care of myself, I was better able to love and take care of others. Instead of feeling like I have nothing left to give because of the weight of depression, anger, disappointment, frustration, regret, guilt, and sorrow I carried around day in and day out, I not only have more of myself to give, but it's a version of myself people actually benefit from now instead of avoid! I still have struggles and stressors in life like anyone else, but I face them with a new hope, strength, confidence, and resolve that I didn't have before. In addition to those in my daily life, I've been able to help countless others CHOOSE THE CHANGE in their own lives, take control of their lives and health, and lose weight while gaining their lives back! As I've said, this is so much more than a physical journey. This CHOICE to change your life will influence every facet of your life and those around you (ones you know and even those you don't) for the better.

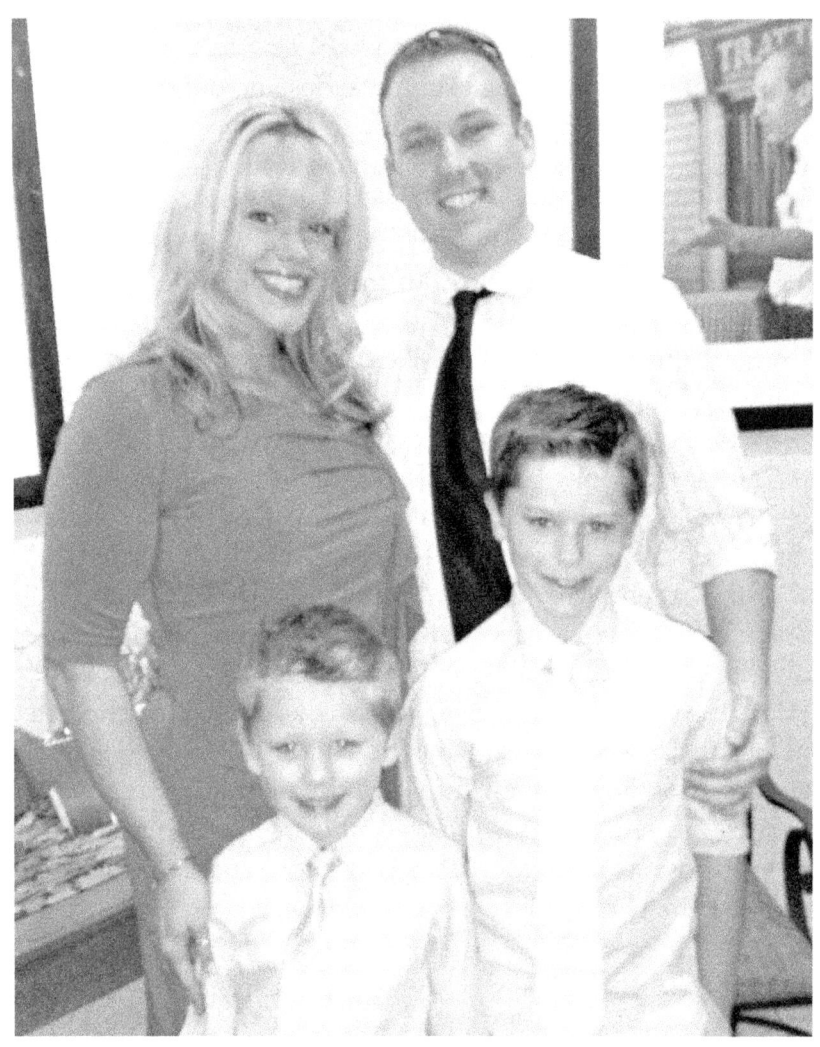

The Donahoo Family, May 2013

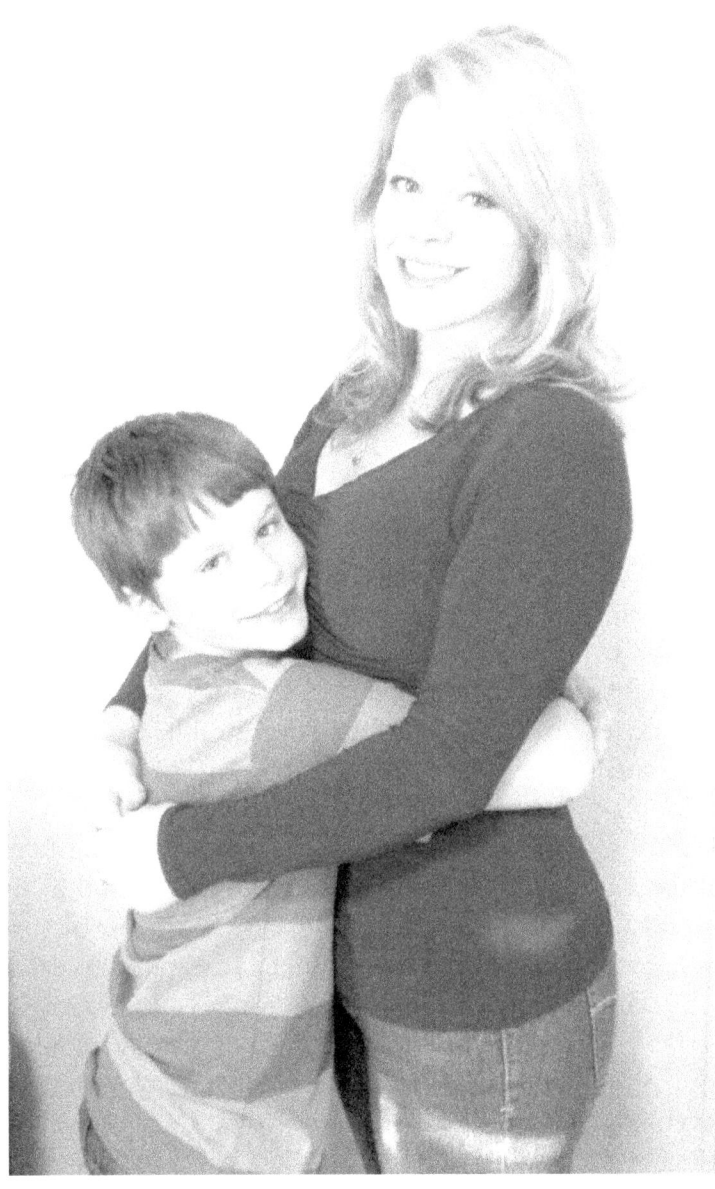

Little moments along my journey like having my eldest jump back in shock when he was finally able to reach his arms all the way round me in a hug were the biggest and most cherished ones, not always just the number on the scale.

After having my two sons then gaining and losing my weight, I was left with some sagging skin around my abdomen and a deflated, sagging chest. I tried everything I could to work off my "mommy tummy" on my own through exercise and nutrition, but nothing changed it. My abdominal muscles had split apart from my pregnancies, and excess skin just doesn't go away on its own. You can see from my before and after photos that I had abdominal definition even with the excess skin – this was not for lack of trying. After keeping my weight off for over a year and a half, and when my husband and I felt we were financially able, I began to search out a plastic surgeon. I had very strict criteria, and did a lot of research on my own and got referrals from others before choosing my doctor. I was planning on a major surgery and results obviously needed to be the best, so I needed the best surgeon working on me. I chose Dr. Nathan Patterson of Patterson Plastic Surgery in Gulf Breeze, Florida for my procedures. He came with stellar reviews and referrals publicly and personally, and from my initial consult and every visit thereafter, I've felt comfortable and confident (before and after my surgery). I chose to have an abdominoplasty (tummy tuck), mastoplexy (breast lift), and augmentation (implants). Although the surgery was fairly recent and I'm still healing, I'm in love with my results and the "before and after." Dr. Patterson and his entire team are just of superior expertise and have held my hand walking me through each step of the entire process (before, during, and after) in a comfortable, kind, and confident manner. I could not recommend a better surgeon and team for any type of personal improvement surgery.

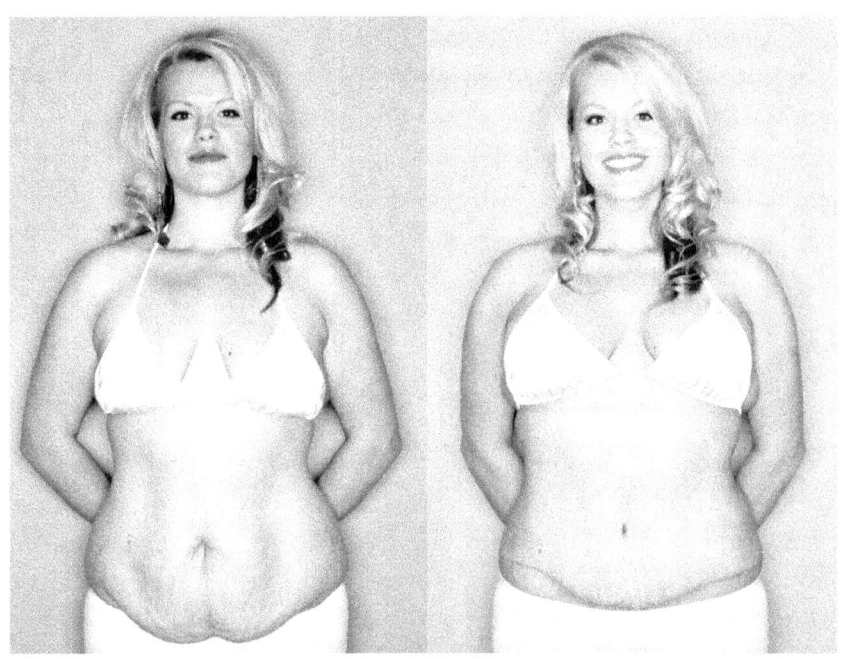

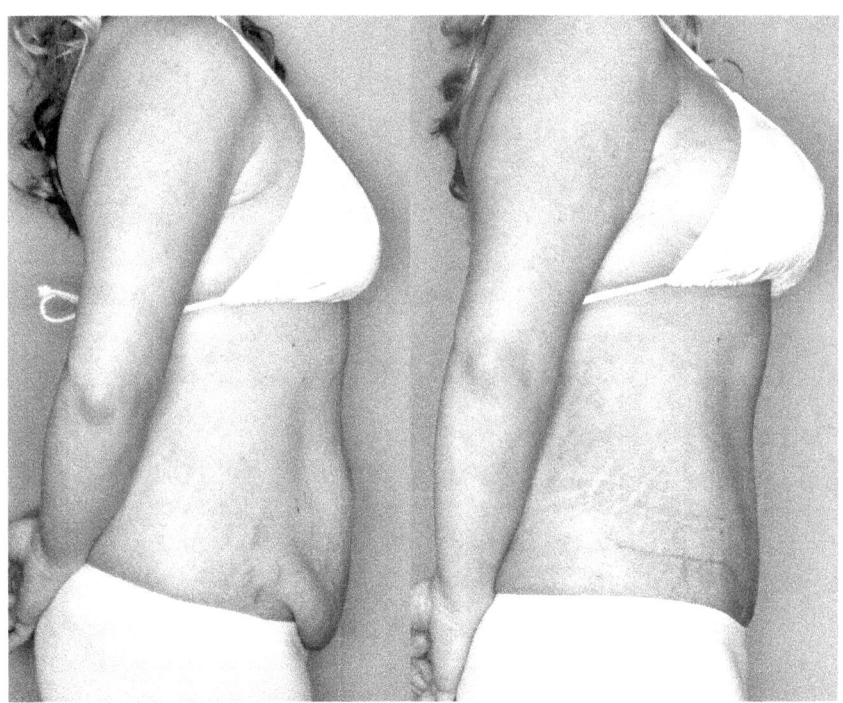

Before & After: Abdominoplasty, Mastoplexy, & Augmentation
by Dr. Nathan Patterson, Patterson Plastic Surgery

I started off slow in my journey. This new lifestyle and the weight loss was not something that just happened overnight. It took me about 20 months to lose all my weight, and I've kept it off because I made this a lifestyle. It's not about total deprivation from foods you enjoy, but modification where you can, and moderation (less of it, less often). Too many times, people think the weight should come off faster, and get discouraged when it doesn't. Keep this in mind in those times: If you're losing the weight faster than you gained it, you're doing phenomenally! Slow and steady is better on this journey, and will make your new lifestyle and weight much easier to maintain after you hit your goal weight. I worked each small change into my life, and they all added up to get me to where I am now. This is a life-long process. I know I will never be perfect, but as long as I am continually improving in some way, I count myself and my life as a SUCCESS.

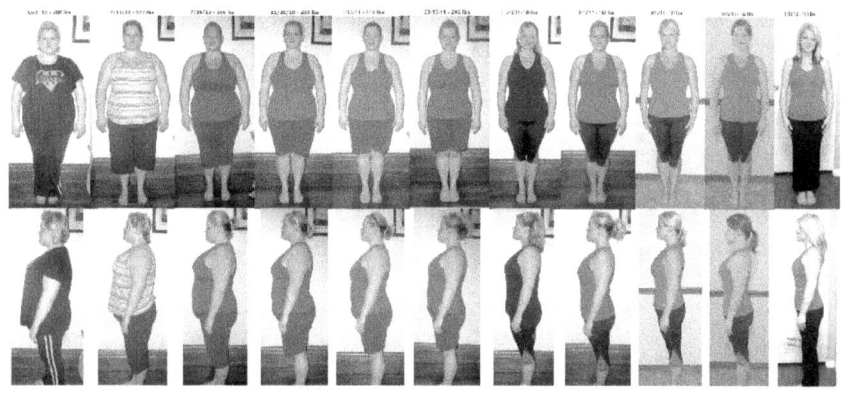

Weight Loss Progression from June 2010 – March 2012
Lost: 137 lbs, over 100", and 11 sizes

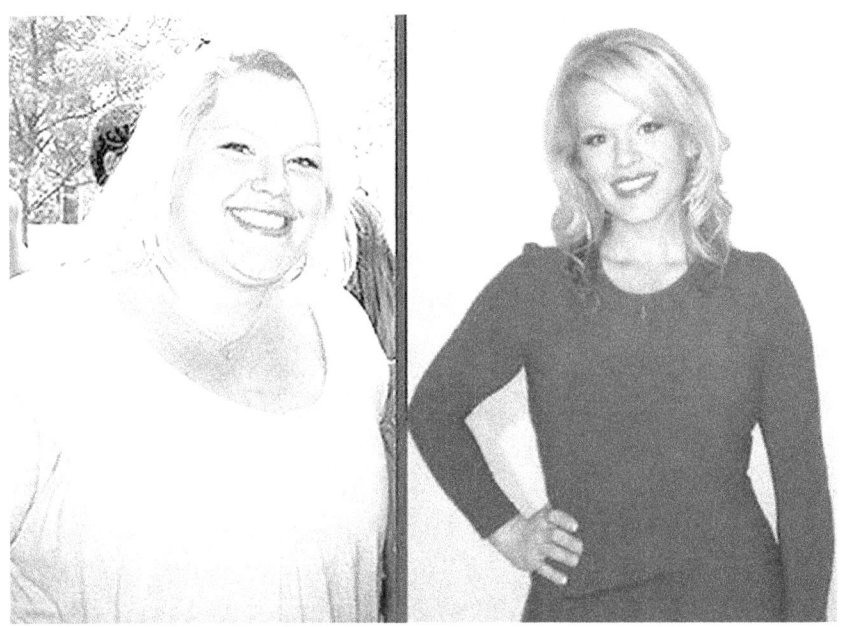

Before & After losing 137 lbs, over 100", and 11 sizes

ASHLEY DONAHOO

3. NUTRITIONAL INFORMATION: FIGHT THE YO-YO!
Why you need to eat to lose.

Growing up, I saw tons of women in my life try to starve off weight. They'd eat less than a bird (and not very appetizing foods at that), and call it "dieting." They'd maybe lose a little weight, then get frustrated, binge, and/or go back to their "normal" eating and gain it back and then some, then start the process all over again. This is what the vast majority of us were raised to think we have to do to lose weight. But guess what? It's WRONG. It's just not that simple, and clearly it doesn't work long term, hence the term "yo-yo dieting." When I decided to lose my weight and change my life, I refused to be a "Yo-Yo Dieter." When trying to lose weight, there are a lot of factors that go into it, but the biggest and most important one is making sure you're eating the right amount of calories (and eating balanced; see Chapter 5). If you drop your calories too low, there are a lot of issues you'll run into – not the least of which is that it's really unhealthy and not maintainable for life. So why doesn't dropping your calories really low work?

Imagine your body having a mind of its own (because it kinda does). When you drop your calories too low, your body starts to "think" you're starving and kicks in its survival mechanism. So the way it combats this is to start trying to store all/ most of the food you DO eat instead of processing and releasing it normally. This causes an increase in fat storage (this is bad). Instead of using those stores for energy (i.e. burning calories), it holds onto them as much as possible and you start feeling weak and tired. Any weight you DO end up losing is not lost through your efforts per se, but by your body literally "eating" its own muscle (yes – this really happens). If you keep your calories too low for too long, eventually your metabolism will slow so much that you plateau and it'll seem like no matter what you do, you just can't lose anymore. This is because your body is in "starvation mode" and is refusing to let go of any fat. So instead of gaining muscle and losing fat, you're losing muscle and gaining fat – this is also bad and the opposite of what you want. I promise your body's ability to hold onto those fat stores will probably outlast your will to starve off the weight (not to mention if you want to keep it off, say goodbye to ever eating "normally" again) – this is a ridiculously frustrating place to be in. At this point, you've trained your body to store and lower your metabolic levels, so when you start "eating normally" again, you gain the weight back and then some because you've wrongfully trained your body by eating too little when losing the weight. This is exactly how "Yo-Yo Dieters" are born.

When you throw in exercise on top of a low-calorie diet, you're asking for double the trouble. You're increasing the stress on your body, but not feeding it near enough to work properly, so your body goes into complete crisis mode. Your metabolism slows to almost a halt, and you put a severe strain on your major organs because you're depriving them of the nourishment they need. The more active you are, the more you need to eat – period. Think of professional athletes and how much they eat, especially when training (we're talking thousands of calories a day) to compensate for the calories they're burning through exercise to keep their bodies working well and to stay healthy and strong.

To lose weight healthily, you want to keep your metabolism burning and make sure you're burning fat and losing at a good pace. How do you do that? Look at your metabolism as a fire: you have to continually feed and poke a fire to keep it burning big and bright, right? Your metabolism is the same way – you have to keep feeding (nourishing) yourself in order to keep your metabolism running at full speed. I encourage people to eat breakfast, a morning snack, lunch, and afternoon snack, and dinner – and if you have enough calories left at the end of the day (hopefully you do), then an evening snack as well. This trains your body and metabolism to expect food at certain times and lets it know that you ARE feeding it, so there's no reason to "think" it's starving. After you do this for a few days, you'll notice you are getting hungry at those times – that means the "training" is working and your metabolism has picked up the pace! You keep that fire burning bright by making sure you're eating enough to maintain health and support your body and energy levels, but low enough so that you lose weight. I refer to this as the Magic Zone. This number will be a little different for everyone because a lot goes into how much a person should eat (age, height, weight, activity level, genetics, etc). (See the info on how to figure out your calorie goal in Chapter 4.)

Another reason not to drop your calories too low is because as you lose weight, you will have to adjust that number along the way (especially if you have a lot of weight to lose). A calorie goal is often a moving target along the journey of a large weight loss. The less you weigh, the less calories you need to maintain your weight, so the less calories you can consume to lose. This is also one reason I tell people to start with a light exercise regimen; the more you lose, the less you will be able to eat unless you increase your workouts/ intensity/ time. So in order to eat enough to not feel like you're starving, you need to pick up your workouts some (not past a maintainable level of course) as you progress in your journey. Leave room to grow, so to speak. Also, the lighter you are, the less calories you will burn when working out. It's all about finding a balance between the two (food and exercise) and constantly evaluating and making sure you're on the right track. You need to find that balance and know in the beginning that you will have to change things along the way.

Something I insist for people to consider is the long-term as well as the short term. Think about the long-term when it comes to calories, weight, and your lifestyle. Is what you're doing maintainable for the rest of your life? If you're eating too few calories the answer that is "No." If you're working out for hours a day, that answer is also, "No." There's only so long you will be able (and willing) to literally starve yourself and/or workout for hours every day. So focus on eating healthily and having a great balance in your life when it comes to food and exercise. Like I said above, this is a moving target because as you lose, you WILL have to adjust things to keep losing. THEN when you're ready to maintain your new weight, that will be a whole new adjustment. So think longer-term when it comes to calories and exercise.

If you need to raise your calories, I realize this is probably a scary prospect for you. No one wants to GAIN weight while they're trying to lose, and a 1-2 pound increase can be very frustrating, I know. Truthfully, you MAY see a slight bump in the scale over the first few days – but DO NOT FREAK OUT about this! Let me explain: Your body is still in storage mode (from you starving it), and until it realizes you're not going to starve it anymore, it'll keep storing. But if you STICK WITH

IT, your body will adjust to the new number and it'll be much happier with that, your metabolism will increase, and you'll start losing again. Anytime you change your calorie goal, give it at least two weeks (I'd prefer 3-4) to let your body adjust. I know this can be frustrating to have to wait, but you just can't make your body respond any faster than it will on its own. TRUST ME, though, once your body adjusts to this number, you will feel SO much better, you'll be healthier, have more energy, AND the weight WILL start coming off if you hit the right number (PLUS the weight will be much easier to KEEP off after you hit your goal)!

This whole journey is about changing your mindset about a lot of things. This journey is so much more mental and emotional than it is physical. This new way of looking at food is part of this journey. Too often, people see food as "good" or "bad," but that's just not the case and not helpful in this journey. Look at food as your body's fuel. Some foods do not contribute to your health or help your weight loss journey, and some do. NO foods are totally off limits, but there are foods (high fat, processed, high sugar, fast foods, etc) that you should limit in your servings and frequency. You have to learn how to nourish your body properly in order to be successful at this and maintain a healthy lifestyle for the rest of your life. Again – it's all about finding that BALANCE.

Remember: This is NOT just a "diet" to lose weight – it's a healthy lifestyle that you're learning and working on – and balancing calories is a big part of that! You CAN do this – one step, one choice at a time! Get the right calorie goal and nourish yourself properly and this journey will be a whole lot easier for you in the short and long terms. Fight the "Yo-Yo" by making healthier choices and making it an overall lifestyle.

4. NUTRITIONAL INFORMATION: FINDING THE MAGIC ZONE
Figuring Out How Many Calories to Eat

1. Figure out our Basal Metabolic Rate (BMR): How many calories you would burn if you literally lay around all day – what your body needs just to function properly.
    a. Women: BMR = 655 + (4.35 x weight in pounds) + (4.7 x height in inches) - (4.7 x age in years)
    b. Men: BMR = 66 + (6.23 x weight in pounds) + (12.7 x height in inches) - (6.8 x age in year)
    c. There are tons of free BMR calculators available online that will do the calculations for you.

2. Use the "Harris Benedict Formula" to figure out how many calories you would have to eat to MAINTAIN your weight based on your current activity level. Multiply your personal "BMR" by the appropriate number below based on your activity level:

    a. Sedentary (little or no exercise) : Calorie-Calculation = BMR x 1.2

    b. Lightly active (light exercise/sports 1-3 days per week) : Calorie-Calculation = BMR x 1.375

    c. Moderately active (moderate exercise/sports 3-5 days per week) : Calorie-Calculation = BMR x 1.55

    d. Very active (hard exercise/sports 6-7 days per week) : Calorie-Calculation = BMR x 1.725

3. To figure how many calories to eat to LOSE weight:

    a. Multiply your "Harris Benedict" number by 7.

    b. Use these guidelines:

        i. If you have 10 lbs or less to lose, subtract 1750 to aim to lose .5 lb a week.

        ii. If you have 11-30 lbs to lose, subtract 3500 to aim to lose 1 lb a week.

        iii. If you have 31-49 lbs to lose, subtract 5250 to aim to lose 1.5 lbs a week.

        iv. If you have 50-84 lbs to lose, subtract 7000 to aim to lose 2 lbs a week.

        v. If you have 85+ lbs to lose, subtract 8750 to aim to lose 2.5 lbs a week.

    c. Divide that number by 7 to get how many calories you should eat per day to lose weight.

As you lose weight, you need to revisit this chart and reevaluate how much you are eating. Weight loss will naturally slow as you have less to lose. That is healthy and perfectly okay. This will also help you keep it off once you enter maintenance.

5. NUTRITIONAL INFORMATION: EATING BALANCED & MACRONUTRIENTS

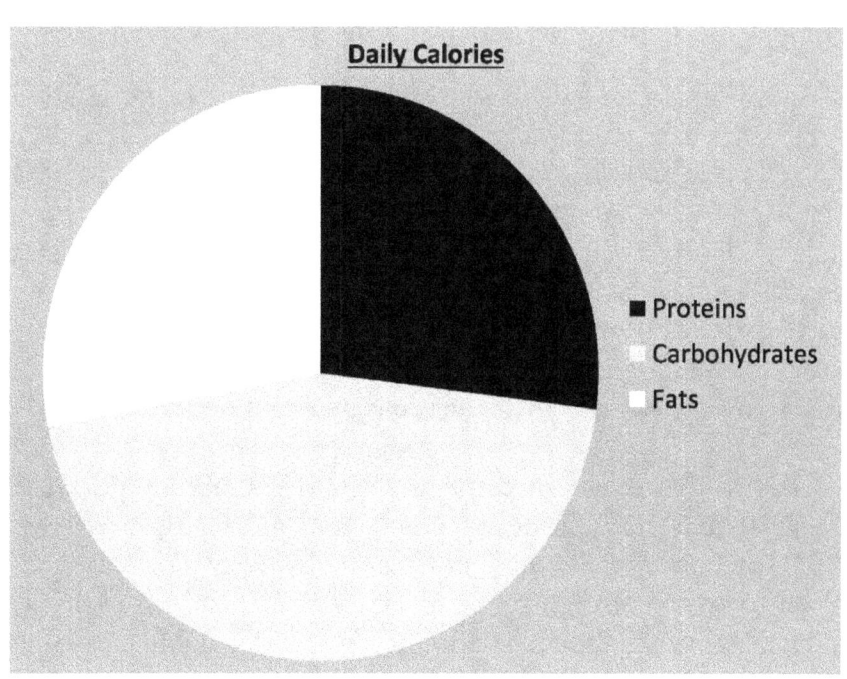

Your daily calorie intake is made up of three Macronutrients: Carbohydrates, Proteins, and Fats. Your body needs ALL of these in order to function properly, and reach and maintain optimum health (including a healthy weight). The pie graph at the beginning of this chapter shows about how much of each macronutrient your daily calories should consist of. Your caloric breakdown of macronutrients should be: 40-50% Carbohydrates, 20-30% Proteins, and 20-30% Fats. This section of the Guide will discuss each macronutrient, how they each interact with the others, how your body uses each, and why they're all important to your weight loss journey and your overall health.

CARBOHYDRATES

Carbohydrates (i.e. "carbs") are often looked at and referred to like they're evil or bad for you. The truth is: THEY'RE NOT! Your body needs carbohydrates all the way down to the cellular level to function properly. Low-carb diets have been linked to several health problems, too. The USDA guidelines actually suggest that you get 45-65% of your calories from carbohydrates! Carbs are one of the three macronutrients (the other two are proteins and fats) that your body needs to function properly and to achieve and maintain optimum health.

Does that mean all carbs are "good"? Certainly not. The foods that have high sugar content and are highly processed (did someone say "doughnut"?) are obviously not nearly as good for you as carbs from vegetables and fruits, for example. Whole grains are also really good for you and should be eaten in moderation (like all things).

So what exactly ARE carbohydrates and how does our body use them? Carbohydrates are the main source of energy for our bodies, and our bodies have an easier time turning carbohydrates into fuel for energy than any other nutrient. Carbohydrates are made up of sugars, fiber, and starches, and can be found in a plethora of foods, including (but not limited to): fruits, vegetables, grains, rice, dairy, legumes, or any food that contains sugar, fiber, or starch.

Further, ALL of the tissues and cells in our body can use the fuel from carbohydrates for energy. Carbohydrates are needed for your central nervous system, kidneys, brain, and muscles (including your heart) to function properly. Your digestive system also relies heavily on carbs for proper functioning. This is where "fiber" comes into play.

I'm sure you've heard a lot about getting "high fiber" in your diet. Fiber refers to carbs that are non-digestible by our bodies. This is actually a GOOD thing. Fiber helps "move things along" in your digestive tract and promotes a healthy "flow" in your digestive tract, and helps your body function more efficiently overall. Carbs also provide essential nutrients to promote good bacteria in your intestines in a way that proteins and fat do not. This helps keep you healthy by increasing the good bacteria to "fight off" the bad bacteria (which equals a lower chance of getting sick by promoting a better immune system).

Low-fiber diets have been linked to health issues like constipation and hemorrhoids and to dramatically increase the risks of some cancers – like colon cancer. Conversely, HIGH fiber diets have been shown to lessen the chance of heart disease, obesity, cancer, AND people with high fiber diets typically have lower cholesterol. Higher fiber and healthy carbs in your diet also help in balancing a healthy blood sugar.

While it is true that your body will also convert proteins and fats into energy if forced to, I am still a supporter of having HEALTHY carbohydrates in your diet. You may benefit from lowering your carbohydrate level from the "recommended" amount, since the recommended amount is a little high in my opinion. However, this is something for you to discuss with your doctor since every person's dietary and health needs do vary some. I personally certainly do not recommend or support "low-carb" diets in any form, though.

In recent years, there has been more and more research done on the harm of low-carb diets in the short and long term. Some research has even begun to support a relationship between low-carb diets over the long-term to Alzheimer's and Dementia because of the serious lack of vitamins and minerals caused by low-carb diets that may cause shrinking of the brain and its cells. Also, if you completely cut out carbs (or have them too low), your body will start using your muscle as fuel (i.e. "eating" its own muscle) before it starts utilizing fats – which is the OPPOSITE of what you should want to do. You want to build muscle and lessen fat, not the other way around. Additionally, trying to force your body to use fats, and especially protein, for a fuel source instead of carbs (by cutting your carbs too low) puts a large strain on your kidneys and liver because they have to work overtime to get energy from those sources instead of from carbs. So once again – it's all in the right BALANCE of the macronutrients that will lead to ultimate nourishment and health.

There is a lot of "sciency" and complicated research articles, news stories, books, and rumors out there on carbs and why our bodies need (or don't need) them, more in-depth break-downs of carbs, etc all over if you're interested – feel free to do the research (but keep in mind you will find conflicting things about just about everything – so be wary of your sources and make sure they're trustworthy). I try to keep the information as simple and easy to understand as possible. SO – here are the basics for carbs as far as I'm concerned:

1. Do NOT cut out carbs or cut them too low.
2. Aim for about 40-50% of your calories to come from "good" carbs
3. Your carbs should mainly be from these types of sources:
   a. Fruits & Veggies
   b. Good veggie sources: Sweet potatoes, carrots, green leafy vegetables, etc.
   c. Whole Grains (i.e. whole/ multi grain breads, cereals, pastas, brown rice, quinoa, whole wheat flour, etc)
   d. Beans and legumes
   e. Unprocessed/ whole foods that naturally have carbs (the less processed it is, the better for you!)
4. Focus on getting a good amount of fiber daily to reap all the health benefits (but if you're following #3, then this should come automatically).

So – for all your carb-lovers out there, FEAR NOT! You do NOT have to give up carbs to lose weight and have a healthy lifestyle! Lord knows I would never have stuck with a low-OR-no-carb diet if I had to in order to lose weight! Just redirect your carbs to come from healthy sources – like those listed above. Focus on eating in a balanced and healthy way, and you'll be fine. Then, for those not-so-healthy carbs (i.e. fast food, desserts, etc), you focus on modification where you can, then moderation (eating less of it less often). Set realistic goals, track your food, make sure you're getting balanced amounts of the three macronutrients (fats, carbs, and proteins), and exercise – it REALLY IS a fail-proof plan!

PROTEINS

Most people know that protein is good for you and that you need it for survival. But do you know WHY? How does your body use protein? What types of foods should you get your protein from? Protein is a macronutrient (like fats and carbohydrates) that is essential to your body's proper functioning and optimum health. The USDA recommends that 10-35% of your calories come from proteins. This amount, in proper balance with your fats and carbohydrates, will promote the best health.

Your body uses proteins in every function of your entire body down to the cellular level. In fact, your DNA is made up of proteins and your cells' nuclei need protein to exist! According to www.eatbalanced.com, "Enzyme proteins break down food for absorption; to regulate the entry of nutrients through cell walls, and the removal of waste-products; to grow, develop, move, reproduce." I'd say that makes protein pretty darn important to your body – just like the other two macronutrients.

There are many other ways your body uses protein that are just as important, though. Your muscles, for example, are mostly composed of protein. Your bones, ligaments, tendons, and joints also are greatly comprised of proteins. Therefore, protein supports your physical movement as well as internal functioning. Collagen, a type of protein used in the aforementioned parts of your body, is also important for your skin and it's elasticity and youthful appearance (like healthy fats). Your hair and nails are also mostly protein (keratin)! Protein is ALL OVER your body!

Having a healthy balance of protein also helps keep you "flushed" out and helps prevent bloating and water retention.

Antibodies (the little guys released by cells to fight off germs and foreign substances) are also made up of proteins! Essentially, in almost every way possible, having the right kinds of proteins in the right amount is VERY important for overall health and proper bodily functioning!

The McKinley Health Center of the University of Illinois (http://www.mckinley.illinois.edu/) attributes protein to be essential in the following:

- "Growth (especially important for children, teens, and pregnant women)
- Tissue repair
- Immune function
- Making essential hormones and enzymes
- Energy when carbohydrate is not available
- Preserving lean muscle mass"

While protein CAN be used for a type of energy source, it is not wise to rely on it heavily for energy – it just won't work well, truthfully. When your body attempts to use protein as a fuel source, it actually breaks down the protein to a carbohydrate form – this takes a lot of energy to do, but it also is not as complete a fuel as if you had healthy carbs and fats contributing to your energy source. Your body has a really hard time using protein as energy, and there are SO many other functions (listed above and then some) that your body needs protein for, that it can actually be counterproductive and even harmful to try to make your body use protein for energy. Simply put, according to www.rawfoodexplained.com:

> "It is for this reason that the popular high-protein, low-carbohydrate diets result in weight loss and also why they are dangerous. Since the body has to expend so much energy in converting the excess protein into the needed

carbohydrates for fuel, a net loss occurs in the body and the dieter loses weight. At the same time, he also places a heavy burden on his kidneys to eliminate all the uric acid generated by this protein breakdown and simultaneously overworks an already exhausted liver."

Proteins from animal meat and proteins from plants are also different in their functions and how our body uses them. For example, animal proteins contain enzymes and amino acids that plant proteins do not. Animal proteins are considered "high-quality proteins" because our bodies are more accustomed to those types of proteins than plant-based proteins (we are animals, after-all). Plant-based proteins are also good in their own ways though, because they typically contain low amounts of fat, and their fats are good fats (see the section in this chapter on fats for more info). Therefore, it's important to make sure you're getting a balanced amount of proteins from various sources in order for your body to glean all the benefits of different types of protein.

So now that you know all about why we need protein and what our bodies use it for, what foods should you aim to get your protein from?

- Lean meats (poultry, fish, lean cuts of beef, etc)
- Dairy & Eggs (milk, cheese, etc)
- Nuts, Beans, and legumes (peanuts, soy, almonds, etc)

Remember that it's all about BALANCE. All three macronutrients in this chapter (proteins, fats, and carbohydrates) are important to your entire body and overall health. Finding the right types of all three macronutrients and getting the right portions of all three is something you can and will learn through education and trial and error. Tracking your food is a BIG part to figuring out proper nutrition, and seeing it right there in front of you to help you learn right from wrong in your nutritional choices. When you find that right balance for your total calorie intake and personal fitness and health goals, you will be amazed at the difference you feel overall. By having a balanced diet (overall nutrition), you are not just increasing your physical health, but your energy levels will increase, and you will also be more balanced mentally and emotionally. All these things work together to help make the best YOU possible – but you have to do your part. Take responsibility for your nutrition and health and make good choices – it really all adds up to amazing results!

FATS

I know it sounds funny, but even though you may be trying to lose fat from your body, you STILL need fats in your daily diet! There ARE healthy fats and not-so-healthy fats, though. Let me explain what fats are, how your body uses them and why you need then, and what foods provide the best types of fat (i.e. healthy fats). Like everything else in life (and like I've said a thousand times and will continue to say), it's all about finding the right balance! The USDA recommends that 20-35% of your calories come from fats! The important part is knowing the different types of fats, which ones you want and don't want, and where to get it from.

Why is fat important? Fat is the body's most concentrated source of energy – meaning that there is more energy available per gram of fat than any other nutrient, which is why your body stores it (for an energy source). Your body can't process the fat AS easily as carbohydrates, though – meaning it takes more energy to use fats as energy than it does to use carbs. This is one reason alone it's good to have a nice balance of all three macronutrients (proteins, fats, and carbs). Therefore, just like low-carb diets, low-fat diets can cause fatigue and foggy-head syndrome (my own diagnosis – haha), among many other problems. Your body NEEDS balanced amounts of all nutrients to function properly. Children, especially, need a healthy amount of "good" fats to promote proper growth and development – so pay attention, Moms, this info can help your kids, too!

So why exactly do you need fats? How exactly does your body use fat that that makes it SO important to your health? Like the other two macronutrients already discussed, your body uses fats down a cellular level to function like it should. Your body uses fat to "insulate" you and your organs. Obviously having too much "insulation" equals being overweight or, worse, obesity, but your organs DO need to be cushioned as protection to some degree (hence one of the dangers of being underweight). Having a proper amount of fat in your diet has also been shown to reduce those cravings for unhealthy things that are so hard to resist. If you're getting balanced amounts of the things your body needs, then it's less likely to yell at you and "demand" things that aren't good for you – and any cravings you do still get from mental and emotional attachment will be less intense and easier to combat.

Your body also uses fat to insulate your nerves! "Myelin" is made up partly of fats, and it coats your nerves to properly conduct signals from your brain all over your body. I don't know about you, but I'd like to know immediately if I'm in danger of burning myself when I straighten my hair, for example! The connection between your brain and body parts is an ESSENTIAL function in which fat plays a role. Fat is also used by your body as an aid in vitamin and mineral absorption. So if you're not getting enough GOOD fats (keep reading – I'll explain the difference between good and bad fats next), then your body will have a really hard time absorbing other nutrients essential for survival and good health.

Healthy fats also promote healthy skin and hair! Want some glorious locks and clear, youthful-looking skin? Making sure you're getting enough healthy fats (in a balanced way) is a good way to help with that! Fat helps maintain cell membranes (the outer portion of a cell), and helps a cell import good things and expel bad things or "waste" in a healthy way. The healthier your cells and the better they are able to function, the better your whole body will function (again – this goes back to eating all the macronutrients in a balanced way).

Finally, there is a plethora of emerging research that fat (along with an overall healthy balanced diet) may play a large role in the production of endorphins (the "feel good" chemicals in your brain)! So having a balanced amount of fats may not only help you physically, but it could definitely be helping you mentally and emotionally too! It really is amazing how healthy, balanced eating can have such a huge impact on your emotional and mental well-being in addition to physical health (my story of overcoming depression through proper nutrition and exercise is a testament to that)! So, essentially, you're doing WAY MORE than "just losing weight" when you eat balanced and healthy – you're helping your brain and emotional stability, too!

Now that you know why you need fat, let me explain the difference between good fats and not-so-good fats. There are three types of fats: saturated, trans, and unsaturated fats. Look at the nutrition labels of food to see this breakdown and be more aware of what foods have what types of fats.

Saturated fats are those you need to watch carefully, and trans fats you should try to avoid altogether. Saturated and trans fats are factors in and can cause an increased risk of heart disease because your body doesn't process them properly and has a hard time breaking them down. Saturated and trans fats are also stored as that "stubborn" fat that are in certain areas and are harder to get rid of through diet and exercise because your body has such a hard time processing them properly.

Saturated fats are typically found in meats, dairy, and fast foods. Trans fats are typically in baked goods/ desserts, fried foods, and processed foods. So a cheeseburger and fries from the fast food joint down the street is going to be heavy in saturated and trans fats, for example (and obviously those are unhealthy foods, so it makes sense).

Unsaturated fats are the "good" fats. Your body "likes" these fats because they are more naturally occurring and your body has an easier time breaking them down and using them properly. Also, unsaturated fats actually lower the bad cholesterol and help raise good cholesterol, lower your risk for heart disease, and work in all the positive ways listed above (i.e. why your body needs fats). Unsaturated fats are found in good, wholesome foods like avocados, olives (olive oil), nuts, and fish.

Hopefully this has helped you understand that fats, like proteins and carbs, CAN BE good for your body if you're getting the right types from the right sources and in BALANCE with each other and your overall lifestyle. This whole journey is about educating yourself about nutrition and learning how to nourish yourself properly to heal and help your body and promote good health in general. Like the other two macronutrients, fats are an important piece of the puzzle in overall nutrition. So don't look at fat as "bad," because it's actually really good for you in the right format and in the right amount. So go ahead, have a little (unprocessed, preferably homemade) guacamole – it's yummy AND good for you!

6. HEALTHY SWAPS

Instead of:	Eat/ Use:
Bacon, Pork	Turkey Bacon
Bagel	Light Bagel "Thin"
Beef, Ground	Ground Turkey/ Chicken
Biscuit	Whole Wheat Dinner Roll
Bread Crumbs	Plain Oatmeal
Bread, sliced	Whole Wheat/ Multigrain Pita Bread
Bread, sliced	Light/ Whole Wheat Tortilla
Cheese, Cream, regular	Neufchatel Cheese
Cheese, regular	Fat Free/ Light Cheese
Chips, Regular	Baked / Multigrain Chips
Chips, Regular	Pita Slices
Chips, Regular	Unbuttered Popcorn

Instead of:	**Eat/ Use:**
Chips, Regular	Veggies (i.e. baby carrots, snap peas)
Chocolate, Milk	Dark Chocolate
Coffee Creamer	Sugar Free Creamer
Coffee/ Latte Order, regular	Sugar Free, Fat Free Order ("skinny")
Crackers, regular	Rye toast/ baked flatbread
Doughnut, Glazed	Cruller
Egg, whole	Egg White
Flour, White	Whole Wheat Flour
Fried Foods	Grilled or Baked
Fries, Potato	Carrot/ Zucchini/ Sweet Potato Sticks
Fruit, canned/ jarred	Fresh Fruit (OR No sugar added)
Fruit, Dried	Fresh Fruit
Hamburger	Turkey or Veggie Burger
Hash browns	Grits
Hot Dog	Turkey/ Veggie Dog
Ice Cream	Light/ Low Fat Ice Cream

Instead of:	Eat/ Use:
Jelly	No Sugar Added Fruit Preserves
Juices, regular	No Sugar Added Juices
Lettuce, Iceberg	Spinach, Dark Greens ("Spring Mix")
Margarine	Whipped Butter
Mayo	Hummus
Mayo	Mashed Avocado
Mayo, regular	Mayo made with Olive Oil
Meat, Dark sections	White Meat (no skin)
Milk, Regular	Fat Free Skim Milk
Milk, Regular	Unsweetened Almond Milk
Milk, Regular	Light Vanilla Soy Milk
MilkShake	Fruit Smoothie (No sugar added)
Muffin, English (regular)	Light Multi Grain English Muffin
Noodles, Spaghetti	Spaghetti Squash
Noodles, White	Whole Wheat/ Veggie Noodles
Oatmeal w/ sugar/ syrup	Oatmeal with honey & cinnamon

Instead of:	Eat/ Use:
Oatmeal, Instant	Steel Cut Oats
Oil	No Sugar Added Applesauce
Oil, Vegetable/ Lard	Extra Virgin Olive Oil
Peanuts	Edamame
Pizza, Meat Toppings	Veggie Toppings
Pizza, regular	Thin-crust, light cheese pizza
Potatoes, Mashed	Mashed Cauliflower
Potatoes, White	Sweet Potatoes
Pudding, Regular	Sugar Free Pudding
Rice, White	Brown Rice
Rice, White	Quinoa
Rice, White	Couscous
Salad Dressing	Light/ NonFat Dressings OR Vinaigrettes
Sauce, Creamy Pasta	Red Tomato Pasta Sauce
Sausage, pork	Turkey Sausage
Soda	Low Sodium Tomato Juice
Sour Cream, regular	Non-fat/ Light Sour Cream

Instead of:	Eat/ Use:
Sour Cream, regular	Plain NonFat Greek Yogurt
Sugar	No Calorie Sweetener
Syrup, Regular	Sugar Free Syrup
Syrup, Regular	Blended/ Mashed Fruit
Waffles, Regular	Smaller Frozen Buttermilk Waffles
White Bread	Light Multi-Grain Bread
Yogurt, Regular/ Low-Fat	Nonfat Greek Yogurt

7. SAMPLE ONE-WEEK NUTRITION PLAN

(Based on 1500 Calories per Day Goal)

(*Note: Depending on your household's size, you will have leftover/ extra from this week's meal plan to apply to next week's meals, others' meals, lunches, etc)

<u>Every Day</u>:
- 10-12 (8 oz) glasses of water
- Balanced Nutrition (40-50% Carbohydrates, 20-30% Proteins, & 20-30% Fats)
- Weigh/ Measure/ Count food to ensure proper serving sizes

Monday = 1470 Calories

- ❖ Breakfast: 285 Calories
    - o 2 egg whites, 1 turkey sausage patty, 1 slice reduced fat pepper jack cheese, 1 everything bagel thin, 2 tbsp sugar free creamer, & 2 cups coffee
- ❖ Morning Snack: 180 Calories
    - o 1 serving Fat Free Greek Yogurt, 2 tbsp chopped walnuts
- ❖ Lunch: 315 Calories
    - o 1 turkey sandwich (2 slices 90 calorie whole wheat bread, 1 tsp honey mustard, 1 serving deli turkey slices, 1 slice fat free American cheese, lettuce & tomato), 1 small can low sodium tomato/ vegetable juice, & red apple
- ❖ Afternoon Snack: 140 Calories
    - o 1 fiber and protein bar
- ❖ Dinner: 400 calories
    - o 1 serving Ashley's Turkey Stroganoff Casserole, 1 cup cut green beans
- ❖ Evening Snack: 150 Calories
    - o Light Ice Cream Cone

Tuesday = 1448 Calories

- ❖ Breakfast: 285 Calories
    - o 2 egg whites, 2 (frozen) buttermilk waffles, 1 tbsp whipped butter, 3 tbsp sugar free syrup, 2 tbsp sugar free creamer, & 2 cups coffee
- ❖ Morning Snack: 80 Calories
    - o 1 serving Fat Free Greek Yogurt

- ❖ Lunch: 390 Calories
    - o 1 serving leftovers of turkey stroganoff casserole & 1 small can low sodium tomato/ vegetable juice
- ❖ Afternoon Snack: 105 Calories
    - o 1 serving baby carrots, 2 tbsp classic hummus
- ❖ Dinner: 488 calories
    - o 1 serving Ashley's Sweet & Sour Turkey Meatballs, ½ cup brown rice, 1 cup broccoli
- ❖ Evening Snack: 100 Calories
    - o 1 cup mixed berries, 2 tbsp light whipped cream

Wednesday = 1530 Calories

- ❖ Breakfast: 255 Calories
    - o 1 egg, 1 egg white, 1 piece light bread with 1 tsp whipped butter, 2 slices turkey bacon, 2 tbsp sugar free creamer, & 2 cups coffee
- ❖ Morning Snack: 175 Calories
    - o 1 apple with 1 tbsp peanut butter
- ❖ Lunch: 340 Calories
    - o 1 serving light & healthy frozen meal & 1 small can low sodium tomato/ vegetable juice
- ❖ Afternoon Snack: 185 Calories
    - o 1 pear & 1 small light granola bar
- ❖ Dinner: 485 calories
    - o 1 serving Ashley's Turkey Stuffed Poblano Peppers, ½ cup brown rice, spring mix salad w/ tomato & 1 tbsp light raspberry walnut vinaigrette
- ❖ Evening Snack: 90 Calories
    - o 1 light ice cream bar

Thursday = 1445 Calories

- ❖ Breakfast: 340 Calories
  - o 1 serving Ashley's Breakfast Skillet, 2 tbsp sugar free creamer, & 2 cups coffee
- ❖ Morning Snack: 180 Calories
  - o 1 serving Fat Free Greek Yogurt & 2 tbsp chopped walnuts
- ❖ Lunch: 345 Calories
  - o 1 light tortilla wrap with 4 oz of baked chopped chicken breast, ¼ cup reduced fat shredded cheddar, ½ tbsp mayo with olive oil, lettuce & tomato, & 1 small can low sodium tomato/ vegetable juice
- ❖ Afternoon Snack: 105 Calories
  - o 1 serving baby carrots, 2 tbsp classic hummus
- ❖ Dinner: 395 calories
  - o 1 serving Ashley's Tuna Noodle Casserole, spring mix salad w/ tomato & 1 tbsp light raspberry walnut vinaigrette & 2 tbsp reduced fat blue cheese crumbles, 1 cup green beans
- ❖ Evening Snack: 80 Calories
  - o 1 frozen fruit bar

Friday = 1535 Calories

- ❖ Breakfast: 260 Calories
  - o 2 egg whites, 1 light English muffin, 1 turkey sausage patty, 1 slice fat free American cheese, 2 tbsp sugar free creamer, & 2 cups coffee

- ❖ Morning Snack: 160 Calories
  - o 1 serving Ashley's Favorite Snack Greenie
- ❖ Lunch: 340 Calories
  - o 1 serving light & healthy frozen meal & 1 small can low sodium tomato/ vegetable juice
- ❖ Afternoon Snack: 270 Calories
  - o 1 apple with 2 tbsp peanut butter
- ❖ Dinner: 355 calories
  - o 1 serving Ashley's Harvest Turkey & Sweet Potatoes & 2 servings Brussels sprouts
- ❖ Evening Snack: 150 Calories
  - o 1 light ice cream cone

Saturday = 1590 Calories
- ❖ Breakfast: 305 Calories
  - o 1 Ashley's Mini Breakfast Quiches, 1 cup mixed fruit, 2 tbsp sugar free creamer, & 2 cups coffee
- ❖ Morning Snack: 80 Calories
  - o 1 serving Fat Free Greek Yogurt
- ❖ Lunch: 340 Calories
  - o 2 slices light bread – toasted with 4 oz (1 small can) chunk light tuna, 1 tbsp mayo with olive oil, 1 tbsp dill relish, lettuce & tomato, and ½ red apple, & 1 reduced fat cheese stick
- ❖ Afternoon Snack: 140 Calories
  - o 1 fiber & protein bar
- ❖ Dinner: 725 calories
  - o 1 Light Dinner Out/ Ordered In (Restaurant)

<u>Sunday = 1560 Calories</u>

- ❖ Breakfast: 280 Calories
  - o 2 Egg Whites, 1 everything bagel thin, 1 slice fat free American cheese, 2 slices turkey bacon, 2 tbsp sugar free creamer, & 2 cups coffee
- ❖ Morning Snack: 170 Calories
  - o 1 oz. mixed nuts
- ❖ Lunch: 300 Calories
  - o 1 serving leftover Ashley's Turkey Stuffed Poblano Peppers, & 1 small can low sodium tomato/ vegetable juice
- ❖ Afternoon Snack: 105 Calories
  - o 1 serving baby carrots, 2 tbsp classic hummus
- ❖ Dinner: 420 calories
  - o 1 serving Ashley's Crock Pot Apples & Cider Pork Pot Roast, 1 serving sliced new potatoes, 1 cup broccoli
- ❖ Evening Snack: 285 Calories
  - o 1 serving Ashley's Low Sugar Pear Crisp & ½ cup light vanilla ice cream

8. SAMPLE GROCERY LIST

(Based on "Sample One-Week Nutrition Plan," Chapter 7)

*Notes: (1) You will have A LOT leftover/ extra from this list to apply to next week's meals, others' meals, lunches, etc (2) Check your fridge/ pantry first! You probably have some of these items already!

<u>Produce</u>

- 7 apples
- 2 Bartlett pears
- 2 cups mixed berries (your choice: blueberries, blackberries, raspberries, etc)
- 1 tub hummus (plain/ original)
- 2 bags baby carrots
- 4 medium sweet potatoes
- 1 bag of baby spinach
- Spring mix salad
- 2 tomatoes
- 6 poblano peppers

- 1 green bell pepper
- 1 yellow bell pepper
- 1 red bell pepper
- 2 yellow onions
- Sliced button mushrooms
- 1 head iceberg lettuce
- 3 medium Idaho potatoes

Frozen

- Buttermilk waffles
- 1 box light ice cream bars
- 1 box light ice cream cones
- 1 box frozen fruit bars
- 1 bag Frozen Brussels sprouts
- 2 bags frozen broccoli
- 1 bag frozen peas
- 2 frozen healthy meals

Meat

- 1 bag frozen turkey meatballs
- 2 lbs ground turkey
- Extra Lean Boneless Pork Shoulder Picnic Roast (2 lb)
- 2 lb turkey breast fillets – OR – 2lb turkey breast roast
- 1 pkg turkey bacon
- 1 pkg turkey sausage patties
- 1 bag frozen chicken breasts (3 lb bag)
- 1 pkg deli thin sliced turkey breast

Dairy

- 1 pkg fat free American cheese slices
- 1 pkg reduced fat pepper jack cheese
- 1 small bag part-skim shredded mozzarella cheese
- 18-pack eggs
- 1 container whipped (real) butter
- 1 container sugar free coffee creamer
- 1 container unsweetened vanilla almond milk
- 1 bag reduced fat shredded cheddar
- 7 containers fat free greek yogurt
- ½ gallon fat free skim milk
- 1 small container light sour cream
- 1 container reduced fat blue cheese crumbles

Pantry

- 1 loaf light wheat bread (90 calories per 2 slices)
- 1 pack light English muffins
- 1 pack everything bagel thins
- 1 container coffee
- 1 container mayonnaise made with olive oil
- 1 container honey mustard
- 1 pkg fiber and protein bars
- 1 pkg low calorie granola bars (90 calories per bar)
- 1 pkg low sodium vegetable/ tomato juice
- 1 lb bag brown rice
- 2 bags whole wheat wide egg noodles

- 2 cans cut green beans
- 2 cans mixed vegetables
- 1 can sliced new potatoes
- 2 cans black beans
- 1 can fat free cream of celery soup
- 2 cans 98% fat free cream of mushroom soup
- 3 cans no sugar added slice pears (OR 4-5 additional fresh pears)
- 1 bottle light raspberry walnut vinaigrette
- 1 small bag chopped walnuts
- 1 small container mixed nuts
- 1 box ground flaxseed
- 1 container plain oatmeal (quick oats)
- 1 small container peanut butter
- 1 bottle sugar free syrup
- 1 bottle sweet & sour sauce
- 1 bottle extra virgin olive oil
- 1 bottle light soy sauce
- 1 bottle Worcestershire sauce
- 1 bottle ketchup
- 1 container dill relish
- 3 - (4 oz) cans chunk light tuna in water
- 1 small bottle apple cider vinegar
- 1 small bottle light apple juice
- Herbs/ Spices:
    - Allspice
    - Cinnamon
    - Ground cloves
    - Paprika

- o Kosher salt
- o Ground black pepper
- o Minced onions
- o Onion powder
- o Garlic powder
- o Minced garlic
- o Ground mustard
- o Ground ginger
- o Tony Cachere's Cajun seasoning
- o Thyme
- o Light Brown Sugar
- o 1 bag granulated Splenda
- o 1 bag whole wheat flour

9. SNACKS & MEAL SIDES IDEAS

Check labels & measure serving sizes!

Fat Free Greek Yogurt	Toasted Pumpkin Seeds
Mixed Nuts	Low-Fat Ice Cream
Greenie Smoothie	Dried Fruit/ Fruit Crisps & Nuts
Fresh Fruit	Fruit & Yogurt Parfait
Fresh Veggies	Rolled deli sliced meat & cheese
Veggies & Hummus	Yogurt & Nuts
Fruit Smoothie	Sunflower Seeds & Fruit
Sliced block cheese w/ peanut butter	Frozen Fruit Bar
Trail mix (no candy)	Snap Peas & Baby Carrots
Whole Wheat/ Low Sugar Cereal	Low Sodium Tomato Juice & Deli-sliced meat
Rye Toast w/ Neufchatel cheese	Fruit w/ plain Greek yogurt & honey
Olives & Multi-Grain Crackers	Egg whites & whole wheat toast

Cherry Tomatoes & Mozzarella Balls	Raisins & Dried Cranberries
Celery w/ peanut butter (or Neufchatel cheese) & raisins	Hummus w/ Pita slices/ Rye toast
Steamed Veggies	Pretzels & Apple Slices
Green Salad w/ Light Dressing	Edamame (raw or baked)
Reduced Fat Cheese Stick	Veggie Chips/ Straws
Low Fat/ Fat Free Cottage Cheese	Unsweetened Almond Milk w/ Chocolate Protein Powder
Protein Bar	Yogurt & Granola
Sugar Free Pudding	Turkey Jerky
Wheat Crackers & Cheese	Oatmeal, flavored, reduced sugar
Neufchatel cheese w/ fruit or veggie	Granola Bar
Fruit slices w/ peanut butter	Frozen Yogurt
Chickpeas	Sliced Tomatoes w/ Feta
Popcorn (unbuttered) w/ peanuts	Cocktail (cooked/ cold) Shrimp & Sauce
Fiber Bar	Small whole wheat tortilla w/ hummus & bean sprouts
Fresh Fruit & Light Whipped Topping	Baked Apple w/ sprinkled brown sugar & cinnamon
Light & Low Sodium Soup	Fresh Veggies dipped in Light Dressing
Sugar-Free Jello w/ Light Whip Topping	Black Beans & Salsa

10. RECIPES: SPECIAL BREAKFASTS

Check "Servings:" in Recipes for correct servings sizes versus Nutrition Label

Mini Breakfast Quiches

Time: 45 mins
Servings: 6

Ingredients:
4 slice Turkey Bacon, chopped
8 Reduced Fat Crescent Rolls
1/4 cup Fat Free Skim Milk
1 egg
5 large Egg White
1 tsp Spices, Chili Powder
1/2 tsp Coarse Kosher Salt
1/2 tsp Ground Black Pepper
1 tbsp Minced Onion

NUTRITION FACTS	
Serving Size: 1 quiches	
Amount per Serving	
Calories 174	Calories from Fat 78.6
	% Daily Value *
Total Fat 8.73g	13%
Saturated Fat 3.6g	18%
Cholesterol 41.04mg	13%
Sodium 673.38mg	28%
Total Carbohydrate 17.56g	5%
Dietary Fiber 0.15g	0%
Sugars 3.35g	
Protein 9.05g	18%
	Est. Percent of Calories from:
Fat	41%
Carbs	40%
Protein	20%

Directions:
Preheat oven to 375. Cook bacon in pan and set aside (chop up before or after cooking). Spray muffin tin.
Meanwhile, set aside 6 crescent rolls, roll up extra two and cut into 6 even chunks - add each chunk to 1 whole roll for extra dough. Press each roll (and it's extra chunk) into a large circle, then press into muffin tin until you have 6 filled tins. Prebake empty dough cups for approx 5-7 mins.
Meanwhile, combine remaining ingredients with eggs and beat well. (Option: Add in fresh chopped spinach to egg mixture)
After prebaking dough cups and removing from oven, pour egg mixture evenly into each crescent-covered tin. Bake for about 13-15 mins.

Breakfast Skillet

Time: 35 mins

Serving: 1 (double ingredients for 2, etc)

Instructions:
2 large Egg White
1 patty Turkey Sausage
1 medium Idaho Potatoes
1 tsp Olive Oil
1/4 medium Yellow Onions
1/4 large Green Bell Pepper
1/2 cup Sliced Buttons
        Mushrooms
2 tbsp Shredded Reduced Fat
        Cheddar Cheese

NUTRITION FACTS	
Serving Size 1 skillet	
Amount per Serving	
Calories 307	Calories from Fat 103 7
	% Daily Value *
Total Fat 11 52g	17%
Saturated Fat 2 53g	12%
Cholesterol 35mg	11%
Sodium 833 73mg	34%
Total Carbohydrate 34 63g	11%
Dietary Fiber 5 45g	21%
Sugars 8 19g	
Protein 22 93g	45%
	Est. Percent of Calories from:
Fat	29%
Carbs	45%
Protein	29%

Directions:
Heat skillet to medium- med/high. Pour in olive oil (you may use a little more than the 1 tsp to cook in, just pour out and blot as much as possible - it should end up coming out to you consuming only about 1 tsp).

Cut potato into about 1-inch cubes and add to skillet to start cooking. Then cut/ slice up the rest of the veggies as big or small as you want. Dice up sausage patty. Whisk egg whites. Cook potatoes in skillet and stir/ flip for 5-10 minutes (these take the longest). Once they are almost done, put the rest of the veggies in skillet in this order and let them cook before adding the next in order: Peppers, Onions, then mushrooms (different cooking times). Let them get soft (as cooked as you like) before adding the sausage. Let that cook for 2-3 minutes, then add egg whites over all the veggies.

Stir it all together and let the egg whites cook. Sprinkle cheese over the top and let it melt. Then put it all on a plate or in a bowl and ENJOY an awesome breakfast!

Breakfast Casserole

Time: 1 hr 15 mins (total)
Servings: 14

Ingredients:
4 eggs
10 large Egg Whites
12 slices Low Sodium Turkey
          Bacon
3 cups Fat Free Skim Milk
8 slices Delightful 100%
          Multi-grain Bread
1 large Green Bell Pepper
1/2 large Yellow Onion
1 cup Mild Shredded Reduced
          Fat Cheddar Cheese
3 oz fresh Spinach
1 tsp Dry Mustard
1 tsp Paprika
1/2 tsp Salt
1/2 tsp Spices, Ground Black
Pepper

NUTRITION FACTS	
Serving Size: 1 pieces	
Amount per Serving	
Calories 120	Calories from Fat 36.4
	% Daily Value *
Total Fat 4.05g	6%
Saturated Fat 1.3g	6%
Cholesterol 66.79mg	22%
Sodium 406.99mg	16%
Total Carbohydrate 9.49g	3%
Dietary Fiber 1.62g	6%
Sugars 3.48g	
Protein 12.3g	24%
Est. Percent of Calories from:	
Fat	25%
Carbs	31%
Protein	40%

Directions:
Preheat oven to 375F. Spray baking dish with nonstick spray
Cook bacon in pan, then set aside. Dice pepper and onion, then
cook in same pan where cooked bacon (until soft or to desired
texture).
Cut bread slices to about 1" cubes and spread in baking dish.
Chop spinach and cooked bacon and sprinkle evenly in dish
over bread, then evenly sprinkle cooked onions and peppers on
top.

Breakfast Casserole (cont'd)

In large bowl, combine eggs, egg whites, milk, salt & pepper (to taste), and remaining spices/ seasonings in large bowl and blend well. Then evenly pour egg mix into baking dishes over other ingredients.
Bake in preheated oven for approx 30-35 minutes or until set.
Divide into 14 equal servings and serve.
**Option: Cover & refrigerate overnight. In the morning, preheat and bake. Add 10-15 minutes to baking time if refrigerated overnight.

Stuffed Breakfast Crescents

Time: 30-35 mins

Servings: 7

Ingredients:

14 Reduced Fat Crescent Rolls

10 large Egg Whites

8 slices Low Sodium Turkey
        Bacon

1/3 cup Reduced Fat Shredded
        Cheddar Cheese

1/5 cup Fat Free Skim Milk

Directions:

Preheat oven to 450 (check this
per the crescent instructions).
Put parchment paper over
cookie sheet.

NUTRITION FACTS	
Serving Size: 1 stuffed crescents	
Amount per Serving	
Calories 248	Calories from Fat 105.4
	% Daily Value *
Total Fat 11.71g	18%
Saturated Fat 5.14g	25%
Cholesterol 14.43mg	4%
Sodium 646.29mg	26%
Total Carbohydrate 24.6g	8%
Dietary Fiber 0g	0%
Sugars 4.6g	
Protein 12.66g	25%
	Est. Percent of Calories from:
Fat	42%
Carbs	39%
Protein	20%

Cook bacon as instructed, then chop up and set aside. Cook egg
whites with milk (scrambling/ stirring to make fluffy). Mix egg
whites with cheese and chopped bacon. Press 2 crescents
together to seal/ make one larger one. Flatten dough, and
portion egg/ cheese/ bacon mixture into center, then roll
dough over to seal and make a "pocket". Place on cookie sheet
and bake for approx 13 minutes.

11. RECIPES: "GREENIES"

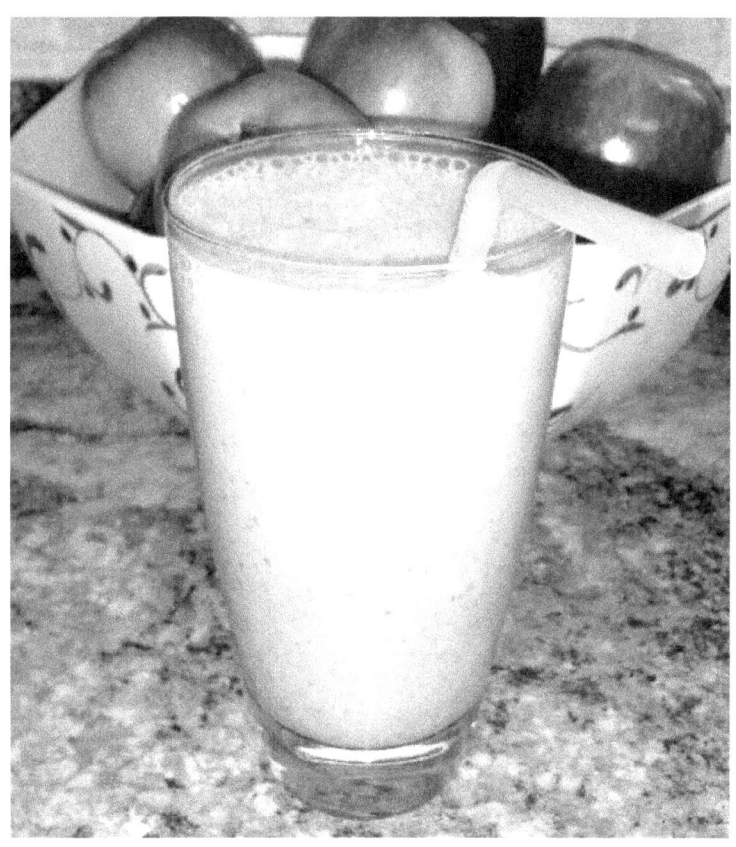

1 serving each

Directions for all: Wilt spinach –OR – kale with about 2-4 tbsp of water in bowl in microwave for approx 30 seconds. Then drain & blend with other ingredients & enjoy.

Berries & Coconut

NUTRITION FACTS
Serving Size: 1 greenie

Amount per Serving
Calories 160   Calories from Fat 36.0

	% Daily Value *
Total Fat 4g	6%
Saturated Fat 0.5g	2%
Cholesterol 0mg	0%
Sodium 152.5mg	6%
Total Carbohydrate 28.5g	9%
Dietary Fiber 6.5g	26%
Sugars 18g	
Protein 5g	10%

	Est. Percent of Calories from:
Fat	20%
Carbs	71%
Protein	12%

Ingredients:
3 oz Baby Spinach
1 cup Frozen Mixed Fruit
1 tbsp Milled Flaxseed
1/2 cup Almond Coconut Milk
8 oz V8 Splash Diet Berry Blend

Berries & Chocolate Protein

Ingredients:
1 1/2 oz Spinach
1/2 cup Frozen Pineapple Chunks
1/2 cup Frozen Blueberries
2 tbsp Ground Flaxseed
8 oz V8 Splash Diet Berry Blend
1 scoops Body Fortress Super
Advanced
Whey Protein Chocolate

NUTRITION FACTS	
Serving Size 1 greenie	
Amount per Serving	
Calories 302	Calories from Fat 65.3
	% Daily Value *
Total Fat 7.25g	11%
Saturated Fat 1g	5%
Cholesterol 47.5mg	15%
Sodium 125mg	5%
Total Carbohydrate 33.01g	11%
Dietary Fiber 9.33g	37%
Sugars 18.17g	
Protein 31.17g	62%
Est. Percent of Calories from:	
Fat	20%
Carbs	43%
Protein	41%

Elvis' Favorite Protein

Ingredients:
1/2 medium Banana
2 large Egg White
1/2 cup Almond Milk
Unsweetened Vanilla
1 tbsp Ground Flaxseed
2 tbsp All Natural Powdered
Peanut Butter
2 1/2 cups Baby Spinach

NUTRITION FACTS	
Serving Size 1 greenie	
Amount per Serving	
Calories 196	Calories from Fat 58.5
	% Daily Value *
Total Fat 6.5g	10%
Saturated Fat 0.05g	0%
Cholesterol 0.1mg	0%
Sodium 344mg	14%
Total Carbohydrate 24.48g	8%
Dietary Fiber 8.1g	32%
Sugars 12.26g	
Protein 16.8g	33%
Est. Percent of Calories from:	
Fat	24%
Carbs	49%
Protein	34%

Strawberry Goodness

Ingredients:
3 oz Baby Spinach
1 cup Unsweetened Almond Milk
1 tbsp Ground Flaxseed
1 container Light & Fit Greek Strawberry
1 1/2 cups Great Value Whole Frozen Strawberries

NUTRITION FACTS
Serving Size: 32 oz

Amount per Serving
Calories 240   Calories from Fat 42.8

	% Daily Value *
Total Fat 4.75g	7%
Saturated Fat 0g	0%
Cholesterol 10mg	3%
Sodium 260mg	10%
Total Carbohydrate 33.5g	11%
Dietary Fiber 9.5g	38%
Sugars 20.5g	
Protein 16.5g	33%

Est. Percent of Calories from:	
Fat	18%
Carbs	55%
Protein	27%

Chocolaty Cherry

Ingredients:
2 tbsp Cocoa (natural, Unsweetened)
8 oz Almond Milk, Vanilla Unsweetened
1 tbsp Ground Flaxseed
1 cup Frozen Dark Cherries
2 1/2 cups Baby Spinach

NUTRITION FACTS
Serving Size: 1 greenie

Amount per Serving
Calories 197   Calories from Fat 59.0

	% Daily Value *
Total Fat 6.55g	10%
Saturated Fat 0.05g	0%
Cholesterol 0mg	0%
Sodium 230mg	9%
Total Carbohydrate 34g	11%
Dietary Fiber 11.6g	46%
Sugars 18.3g	
Protein 6.6g	13%

Est. Percent of Calories from:	
Fat	26%
Carbs	69%
Protein	13%

Peanut Butter Chocolate Cheesecake Protein

Ingredients:
1 tbsp Ground Flaxseed
1 cup Almond Milk Unsweetened Vanilla
2 tbsp 100% Whey Protein
2 1/2 cups Baby Spinach
1/2 tsp Pure Vanilla Extract
1 tbsp Cocoa Powder, Natural Unsweetened
1 tbsp Granular Splenda
2 tbsp All Natural Powdered Peanut Butter

NUTRITION FACTS	
Serving Size 1 greenie	
Amount per Serving	
Calories 235	Calories from Fat 79 0
	% Daily Value *
Total Fat 8 78g	13%
Saturated Fat 0 05g	0%
Cholesterol 34 78mg	11%
Sodium 358 68mg	14%
Total Carbohydrate 17 1g	5%
Dietary Fiber 8 6g	34%
Sugars 2 67g	
Protein 32 14g	64%
Est. Percent of Calories from:	
Fat	33%
Carbs	29%
Protein	54%

Refreshing Icy Pineapple

Ingredients:
2 1/2 cups Baby Spinach
2 cups Pineapple Chunks (frozen)
1 tbsp Ground Flaxseed
1 cup unsweetened almond milk
3-4 Icecubes

NUTRITION FACTS	
Serving Size 1 greenie	
Amount per Serving	
Calories 197	Calories from Fat 45 5
	% Daily Value *
Total Fat 5 05g	7%
Saturated Fat 0 05g	0%
Cholesterol 0mg	0%
Sodium 230mg	9%
Total Carbohydrate 35g	11%
Dietary Fiber 6 6g	26%
Sugars 26 3g	
Protein 4 6g	9%
Est. Percent of Calories from:	
Fat	11%
Carbs	71%
Protein	9%

Ashley's Favorite Snack Greenie

NUTRITION FACTS	
Serving Size: 1 greenie	
Amount per Serving	
Calories 160	Calories from Fat 33.8
	% Daily Value *
Total Fat 3.75g	5%
Saturated Fat 0.25g	1%
Cholesterol 0mg	0%
Sodium 195mg	8%
Total Carbohydrate 17g	5%
Dietary Fiber 4.5g	18%
Sugars 2g	
Protein 16g	32%
	Est. Percent of Calories from:
Fat	25%
Carbs	42%
Protein	40%

Ingredients:
2 cups Baby Spinach
1 tbsp Ground Flaxseed
4 oz Unsweetened Almond Milk Vanilla
8 oz Diet V8 Splash
6 oz fat free greek yogurt

12. RECIPES: DINNERS

If recipe does not call for a serving of green veggies and/ or a carb, add it to the side for a complete meal! Refer to Snacks & Sides List for ideas.

Check "Servings:" in Recipes for correct servings sizes versus Nutrition Label

Turkey Meatloaf

```
NUTRITION FACTS
Serving Size: 1/6 loaf

Amount per Serving
Calories 288          Calories from Fat 110.3

                                    % Daily Value *

Total Fat 12.25g                          18%
    Saturated Fat 3.71g                   18%
Cholesterol 137.5mg                       45%
Sodium 896.67mg                           37%
Total Carbohydrate 10.08g                  3%
    Dietary Fiber 1g                       4%
    Sugars 3.58g
Protein 30.25g                            60%
```

Time: 45 mins
Servings: 6

Ingredients:
2 lb Ground Turkey Meat
¾ cup Plain Oatmeal
5 tbsp Tomato Ketchup
1 tbsp Creole Seasoning
1 egg

Directions:
Preheat oven to 425.
Add oatmeal, 4 tbsp of ketchup, meat, egg, and seasoning and mix well with hands. Spray a bread pan with nonstick spray and spread mixture into pan (or mold into loaf-shape and put on a baking sheet). Top with remaining tbsp of ketchup.
Bake for about 35-40 mins (until browned on top and cooked inside).

Sweet & Sour Meatballs & Rice

Time: 35 mins

Servings: 6 (1 serving = 5 meatballs, 1/5 sauce & peppers, ½ cup cooked rice)

Ingredients:
30 frozen turkey meatballs
1 cup Sweet & Sour Sauce
1 tsp Onion Powder
1 tsp Garlic Powder
1 tsp Ground Ginger
1 tsp Ground Mustard
2 tbsp Soy Sauce
1 tbsp Worcestershire Sauce
1 Yellow Bell Pepper
1 Red Bell Pepper
1 ½ cup (dry) brown rice

NUTRITION FACTS

Serving Size 5 meatballs

Amount per Serving

Calories 473	Calories from Fat 99.0
	% Daily Value *
Total Fat 11g	16%
Saturated Fat 0g	0%
Cholesterol 0mg	0%
Sodium 735.22mg	30%
Total Carbohydrate 60.74g	20%
Dietary Fiber 3.93g	15%
Sugars 17.97g	
Protein 30.22g	60%

Directions:
Prepare rice as directed on packaging. Cut off tops and remove seeds from bell peppers, then slice into strips. Add all ingredients EXCEPT rice to large pan (with about 2/3 cup of water) and stir well. Cook covered on med/high heat, stirring occasionally, for about 30 minutes. You may add ¼ cup water to thin sauce along the way (to get to the desire consistency and avoid burning sauce). Ensure meatballs are thoroughly cooked before serving. Serve meatballs, peppers, & sauce over rice.

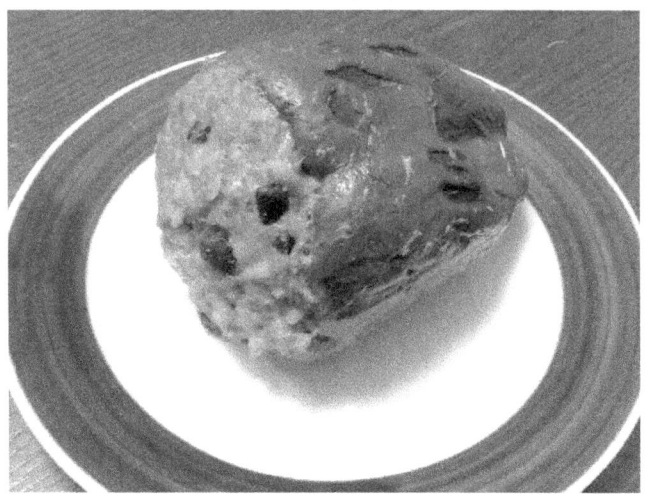

Stuffed Poblano (or Bell) Peppers

NUTRITION FACTS	
Serving Size: 1 stuffed pepper	
Amount per Serving	
Calories 302	Calories from Fat 83.1
	% Daily Value *
Total Fat 9.23g	14%
Saturated Fat 2.84g	14%
Cholesterol 58.33mg	19%
Sodium 837.11mg	34%
Total Carbohydrate 30.45g	10%
Dietary Fiber 6.23g	24%
Sugars 1.42g	
Protein 24.07g	48%

Stuffed Poblano (or Bell) Peppers

Time: 60 mins
Servings: 5

Ingredients:
1 lb Ground Turkey
1 3/4 cups Black Beans
1/2 cup (dry) Brown Rice
¼ cup Plain Instant Oatmeal
3 tbsp Ketchup
1 tbsp Cajun Seasoning
5 Poblano –OR – Large Bell Peppers
1/2 cup Shredded Reduced Fat Cheddar Cheese
1 tsp Extra Virgin Olive Oil

Directions:
Parcook brown rice: Instead of a full cup of water (for half a cup of rice), only use half, then when water is cooked off (about 20 minutes in), remove rice from heat, stir, then use in recipe below. Preheat oven to 375. Spray cooking dish (I use a large rectangle Pyrex dish) with nonstick spray.
Turn on stove burner on high and, using tongs, take each pepper and slightly brown/ blacken outsides (this can also be done on a grill). Cut tops off peppers and remove all seeds and rinds from inside (simple - just use knife to clean around). Wipe outside of peppers with damp paper towel to remove extra charring.
Put turkey, beans, seasonings, beans, rice, ketchup, and crushed crackers in bowl and mix well with hands. Take mixture and firmly stuff peppers well to brim. Place stuffed peppers in dish and cover with aluminum foil. Bake at 375 for about 30 minutes.

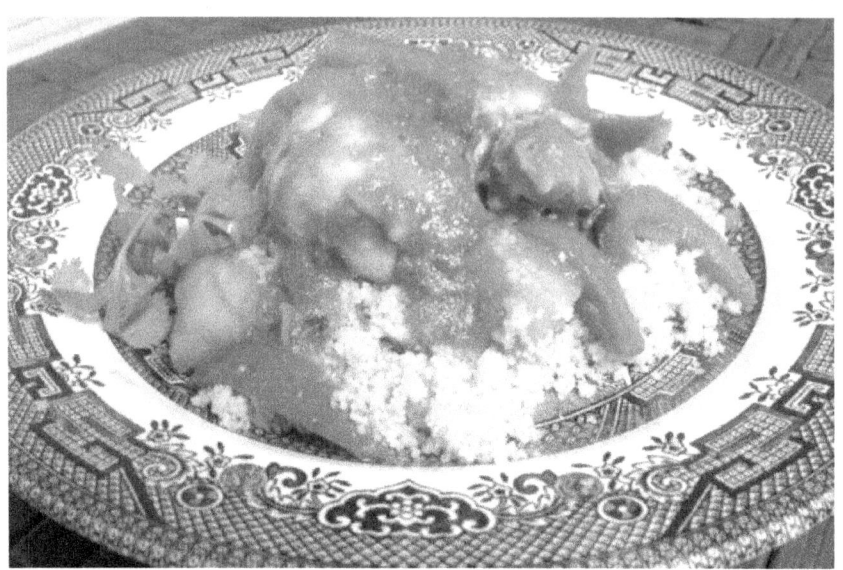

Spicy Ginger Chicken & CousCous

NUTRITION FACTS

Serving Size: 1 chicken breast

Amount per Serving	
Calories 334	Calories from Fat 55.2

	% Daily Value *
Total Fat 6.13g	9%
Saturated Fat 1.79g	8%
Cholesterol 86.25mg	28%
Sodium 832.5mg	34%
Total Carbohydrate 40.4g	13%
Dietary Fiber 3.39g	13%
Sugars 9.02g	
Protein 33.96g	67%

Spicy Ginger Chicken & CousCous

Time: 30-45 minutes
Servings: 6 (1 chicken breast, 1/6th sauce mix,
& ¾ cup cooked couscous each)

Ingredients:
30 oz boneless skinless chicken breasts (6 med)
2 tbsp Salted Whipped Butter
1 medium Red Bell Pepper, Raw, cut into strips
2 medium Green-bell Pepper, cut into strips
1 can (8 oz) Pineapple Chunks in Light Syrup
3/4 cup Picante Sauce
5 sprigs Cilantro, chopped
1 1/2 tsp Ground Ginger
1 1/3 cups (dry) Wheat Couscous

Directions:
Heat butter in large skillet over med-high heat. Add chicken
breasts and cook about 5 minutes on each side until browned.
Remove chicken from skillet and set aside. Meanwhile, cook
couscous as directed on packaging.
To skillet, add pepper strips, pineapple (with juice), picante
sauce, cilantro, salt, and ginger. Cook mixture about 6-8 minutes
until peppers are tender and sauce thickened, stirring frequently.
Return chicken to skillet with mixture, stirring and tossing with
peppers, until heated through.
Serve chicken over couscous.

Stinky 5 Cheese & Pepperoni Pizza

Time: 20 mins
Servings: 3 (cut pizza into 6 slices)

Ingredients:
1 whole wheat pizza crust
1 tsp Extra Virgin Olive Oil
1/2 cup Fire Roasted Pizza Sauce
2/3 cup Finely Shredded Italian Style Cheese
1/4 cup Reduced Fat Crumbled Blue Cheese
1/4 cup Feta Cheese
1 cup Baby Spinach
18 slices Turkey Pepperoni

NUTRITION FACTS

Serving Size: 1/3 pizza

Amount per Serving	
Calories 341	Calories from Fat 102.5

	% Daily Value *
Total Fat 11.39g	17%
Saturated Fat 4.47g	22%
Cholesterol 30.83mg	10%
Sodium 1002.79mg	41%
Total Carbohydrate 41.33g	13%
Dietary Fiber 3.78g	15%
Sugars 4g	
Protein 18.61g	37%

Directions:
Preheat oven to 450.
Brush olive oil on crust, and prebake in oven for about 5 minutes. Remove from oven.
Spread sauce on crust. Add italian blend shredded cheese, then sprinkle on blue cheese. Evenly place spinach all over cheese. Evenly sprinkle feta over top, then evenly space pepperoni over all. Bake for 7-10 minutes or until desired doneness.

Chicken Broccoli Divan Casserole

Time: 30-35 mins
Servings: 4

Ingredients:
20 oz Chicken Breasts, Boneless, Skinless (4 med/lg)
4 1/2 cups Frozen Broccoli Florets
2 tbsp Plain Bread Crumbs
1 tbsp Light Margarine
1 1/4 cups 98% Fat Free Broccoli Cheese
1/3 cup Fat Free Skim Milk
1/2 cup Mild Shredded Reduced Fat Cheddar Cheese

NUTRITION FACTS	
Serving Size 1/4 casserole	
Amount per Serving	
Calories 277	Calories from Fat 58 5
	% Daily Value *
Total Fat 6 5g	10%
Saturated Fat 2 38g	11%
Cholesterol 79 38mg	26%
Sodium 808 36mg	33%
Total Carbohydrate 15 96g	5%
Dietary Fiber 0 88g	3%
Sugars 7 21g	
Protein 39 12g	78%
Est. Percent of Calories from:	
Fat	21%
Carbs	23%
Protein	56%

Directions:
Preheat oven to 450.
Cut up chicken into cubes and cook in skillet.
Spray dish with non stick spray. Place/ Stir broccoli and chicken in 9" pie plate. Stir bread crumbs and butter in small bowl.
Stir soup and milk in small bowl until smooth, then pour over broccoli and chicken. Spread cheese evenly over top. Sprinkle bread crumbs over mixture.
Bake in oven at 450 for about 20-25 mins or until hot and bubbly.

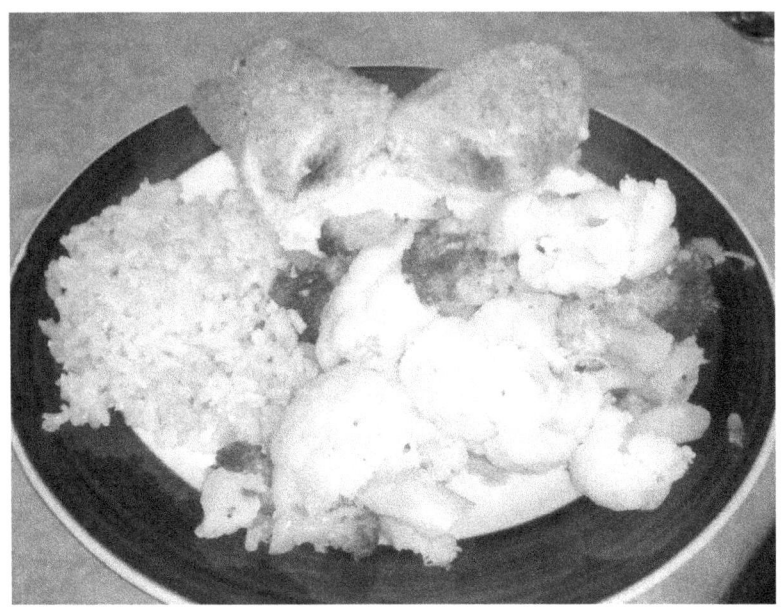

<u>Cheesy Bacon Stuffed Chicken</u>

NUTRITION FACTS
Serving Size: 1 stuffed breasts

Amount per Serving
Calories 272   Calories from Fat 86.6

	% Daily Value *
Total Fat 9.62g	14%
Saturated Fat 4.13g	20%
Cholesterol 106.25mg	35%
Sodium 740.21mg	30%
Total Carbohydrate 8.19g	2%
Dietary Fiber 0.69g	2%
Sugars 1.2g	
Protein 37.38g	74%

Est. Percent of Calories from:	
Fat	7%
Carbs	12%
Protein	54%

Cheesy Bacon Stuffed Chicken

Time: 50-60 mins
Servings: 4

Ingredients:
20 oz Boneless, Skinless Chicken Breast (4 med/large breasts)
4 slices Lower Sodium Turkey Bacon
1 cup Reduced Fat shredded Mexican blend cheese
1/3 cup Plain Bread Crumbs
1 tsp Garlic Powder
1 tsp Onion Powder
1/2 tsp Kosher Salt
1/2 tsp Ground Black Pepper

Directions:
Preheat oven to 425. Spray large casserole dish with nonstick spray.
Mix bread crumbs and spices in pie plate (or other lipped container).
Take long piece of plastic wrap and spray with non-stick spray. Place one breast at a time onto one side of wrap, then loosely cover with other side of sprayed wrap. Take wooden spoon, spatula, can, or any other tool of your choice and beat/ flatten out chicken breast to approx 1/4" thick (careful not to tear sides when flattening). Open plastic wrap, and spray one side of the flattened breast.
Place sprayed-side of breast down into bread crumb mixture. Put 1/4 cup of cheese near one edge (not quite to the end), then top with one piece of bacon (crumble or cut into pieces as you go so you know it's only one piece per breast). Take nearest side, and carefully roll/ wrap breast around filling, tucking in any loose sides that may be spilling out filling. Place in cooking dish. Repeat for all breasts. Bake for about 30-40 mins until completely cooked.

Eggplant Lasagna

Time: 1 hr
Servings: 6

Ingredients:
1 med Whole Eggplant
2 large Egg Whites
1 lb Ground Turkey
1 3/4 cups Ricotta
Cheese (15oz Container)
2 1/2 cups Tomato &
Basil Pasta Sauce
1 tsp Italian Seasoning
1 tsp Garlic Powder
1 1/2 tbsp dried Minced
Onions
1 tsp Coarse Kosher Salt
1/5 cup Shredded Part-
skim Mozzarella
3/4 cup grated Parmesan
Cheese

NUTRITION FACTS
Serving Size: 1/6 lasagna

Amount per Serving	
Calories 328	Calories from Fat 138.8

	% Daily Value *
Total Fat 15.42g	23%
Saturated Fat 7.05g	35%
Cholesterol 101mg	33%
Sodium 977.5mg	40%
Total Carbohydrate 17.73g	5%
Dietary Fiber 3.17g	12%
Sugars 8.57g	
Protein 29.97g	59%

Est. Percent of Calories from:	
Fat	42%
Carbs	21%
Protein	36%

Directions:
Preheat oven to 400. Peel & thinly slice eggplant.
Preheat non-stick skillet and lightly spray with no-calorie non-stick spray. Lightly brown eggplant slices and set aside.
In same skillet, add minced onions, garlic powder, and turkey. Brown turkey over medium-high heat until moisture is gone. Once turkey is browned, add sauce to make meat sauce and bring to a bubble. Allow to lightly simmer for about 3-5 mins, stirring occasionally.
Meanwhile, mix salt, egg whites, and ricotta in a bowl and set aside.

Eggplant Lasagna (cont'd)

Spray a rectangle baking dish with nonstick spray and place ½ of eggplant slices in bottom, covering as much of bottom as possible. Then spread half of ricotta mixture over eggplant, then half of meat mixture on top of that. Then sprinkle 1/4 cup of parmesan cheese over meat mixture. Then evenly place the rest of the eggplant slices, ricotta, then meat in same order. Top with remaining parmesan, then mozzarella cheese.
Place uncovered in preheated oven for about 20 mins until heated through, and top is melted and slightly bubbly.

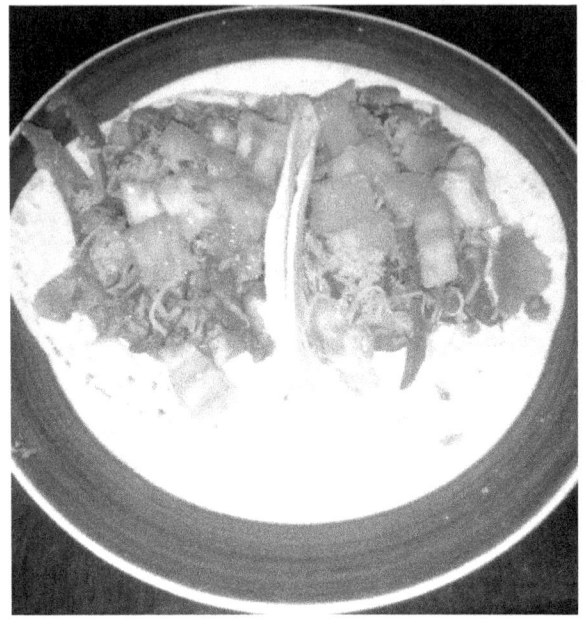

Easy Swai Fish Fajitas

NUTRITION FACTS	
Serving Size: 2 fajitas	
Amount per Serving	
Calories 338	Calories from Fat 102.2
	% Daily Value *
Total Fat 11.36g	17%
Saturated Fat 5.37g	26%
Cholesterol 55mg	18%
Sodium 856.8mg	35%
Total Carbohydrate 34.75g	11%
Dietary Fiber 16.98g	67%
Sugars 9g	
Protein 25.43g	50%

<u>Easy Swai Fish Fajitas</u>

Time: 25 mins
Servings: 4

<u>Ingredients:</u>
1 lb Swai Fillets, cut into 1" chunks
1 large Green Bell Pepper
1 red bell pepper
5 sprigs Cilantro, Fresh
1 medium Yellow Onions
1 medium Tomato Fresh
2 1/2 cups Iceberg Lettuce
2 tsp Chili Powder
1 tsp Minced Garlic
1 tsp Ground Cumin
8 Low Carb Fajita size flour Tortillas
2 tsp Extra Virgin Olive Oil
2 tbsp Lemon Juice
4 tbsp Light Sour Cream
1/3 cup Mild Shredded Reduced Fat Cheddar Cheese

<u>Directions:</u>
Thinly slice up onion & bell peppers (remove seeds first). Chop cilantro. Cut fish into chunks. Chop tomatoes and lettuce.
Heat oil in large skillet to med-high heat. Add pepper and onion slices with chili powder, cumin, and lemon juice, and sauté for 2-3 mins, stirring often, until beginning to soften.
Add chunks of fish to pan, cooking 2-3 minutes per side, until brown on both sides and cooked thoroughly. Meanwhile, gently heat tortillas in microwave, covered with damp paper towel.
Once fish, onions, and peppers are cooked, remove from heat. For each fajita, assemble: spread some light sour cream, add 1 portion of fish with onions and peppers (and some sauce from pans), top with lettuce, tomato, and reduced fat cheese.

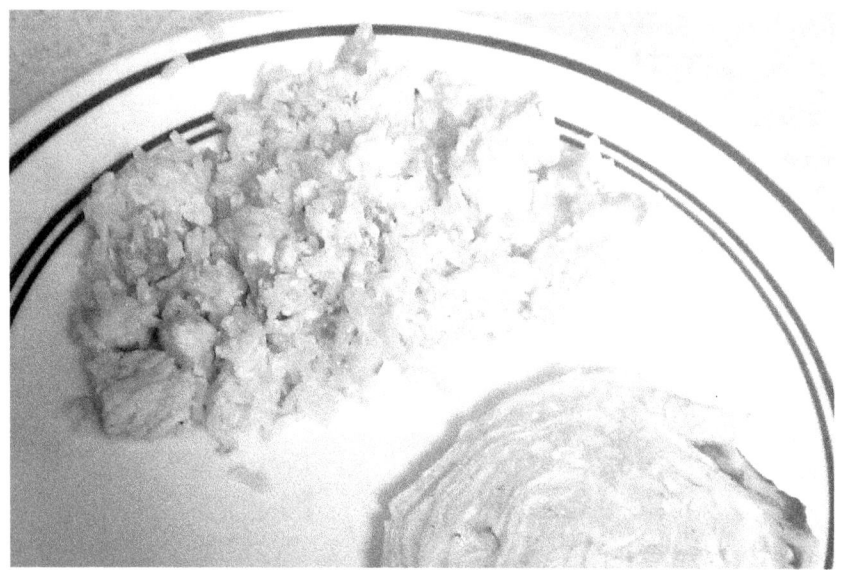

Rice & Turkey Quiche

NUTRITION FACTS	
Serving Size: 1/8 quiche	
Amount per Serving	
Calories 223	Calories from Fat 42.7
	% Daily Value *
Total Fat 4.74g	7%
Saturated Fat 1.83g	9%
Cholesterol 41.94mg	13%
Sodium 356.46mg	14%
Total Carbohydrate 29.58g	9%
Dietary Fiber 2.14g	8%
Sugars 2.05g	
Protein 15.31g	30%

Rice & Turkey Quiche

Time: 25 minutes (not including rice/ turkey cooking/prep)
Servings: 8

Ingredients:
1 1/2 cups (dry) Brown Rice
9 oz Boneless Skinless Turkey Breast
1 tomato, seeded & diced
1 large Green Bell Pepper, seeded & diced
2 tsp dried Basil
1/8 tsp Ground Red Pepper
1/4 cup dried Diced Onions
1/2 tsp Seasoned Salt
1/2 cup Fat Free Skim Milk
2 large Egg White, beaten
1 Egg, beaten
1/2 cup Reduced Fat Shredded Cheddar
1/2 cup Shredded Part-skim Mozarella Cheese

Directions:
Cook rice as directed on packaging, then cool to room
temperature. Back turkey breast and chop into 1/2" chunks.
(These steps can be done the day before for faster prep).
Preheat oven to 375F. Spray 13x9" baking dish with nonstick
spray.
Combine rice, turkey, tomato, onion, green pepper, basil, salt,
ground pepper, milk, & eggs in baking dish. Top with cheeses.
Bake in preheated oven for about 20 minutes, or until knife
inserted in center comes out clean. Cut into 8 equal portions.

Mediterranean Herb Chicken Skillet

Time: 40 mins
Servings: 4

Ingredients:
1 lb Chicken Breasts
(boneless, skinless)
1/4 cup Whole Wheat flour
2 tbsp Extra Virgin Olive
Oil
1 medium Yellow Onion
1 large Green Bell Pepper
1/2 tsp Chicken Flavor
Instant Bouillion Granules
14 1/2 oz Petite Diced
Tomatoes (1 can)
2 tbsp Mediterranean Herb
Seasoning

NUTRITION FACTS
Serving Size: 1/4 skillet

Amount per Serving
Calories 240   Calories from Fat 87.3

	% Daily Value *
Total Fat 9.7g	14%
Saturated Fat 1.5g	7%
Cholesterol 65mg	21%
Sodium 474.6mg	19%
Total Carbohydrate 14.65g	4%
Dietary Fiber 3.11g	12%
Sugars 5.44g	
Protein 25.76g	51%

Est. Percent of Calories from:	
Fat	35%
Carbs	24%
Protein	42%

Directions:
Cut bell pepper into thin strips. Cut onion into 1/2 inch thick
wedges (or use dried minced/ chopped onion). Mix chicken
granules with 1/2 cup of hot water to create a broth. (DO NOT
drain tomatoes from can)
Mix flour and seasoning. Set 2 tbsp aside. Coast chicken breasts
(4) in remaining flour mix.
Heat oil in large skillet on med-high heat. Add coated chicken
and cook about 3 mins on each side to get a crispy outside.
Remove chicken from skillet. Add peppers and onions to skillet.
Cook about 3-5 mins to soften/ cook.
Stir in tomatoes (and juices), broth, and reserved flour mixture.
Bring to a boil, stirring frequently. Add chicken back to skillet.
Reduce heat to low; cover and simmer about 10 mins until
chicken is cooked through. Serve over quinoa, couscous, or
brown rice.

Meaty Mac & Cheese

NUTRITION FACTS

Serving Size: 1 1/3 cup

Amount per Serving

Calories 430	Calories from Fat 133.5

	% Daily Value *
Total Fat 14.83g	22%
Saturated Fat 7.17g	35%
Cholesterol 83.75mg	27%
Sodium 703.33mg	29%
Total Carbohydrate 49.92g	16%
Dietary Fiber 5g	20%
Sugars 6.92g	
Protein 24g	48%

Est. Percent of Calories from:	
Fat	30%
Carbs	46%
Protein	22%

Time: 25
Servings: 6

Ingredients:
1 lb Turkey, Ground
15 oz Macaroni & Cheese (1 standard box)
6 tbsp whipped butter
1/2 cup Fat Free Skim Milk
1 tbsp dried Minced Onion

Directions:
In a large skillet, brown turkey meat with minced onions and drain.
Make Macaroni and Cheese as directed by box in large pot.
Fold turkey and macaroni and cheese in together in pot you made the macaroni and cheese in.
Add any spices you'd like for varying flavors, spiciness, etc.

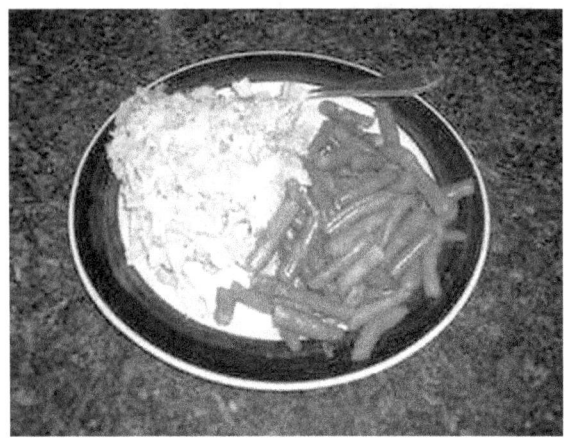

Turkey Stroganoff Casserole

NUTRITION FACTS

Serving Size: 1/6 casserole

Amount per Serving

Calories 359	Calories from Fat 100.0

	% Daily Value *
Total Fat 11.11g	17%
Saturated Fat 3.75g	18%
Cholesterol 107.5mg	35%
Sodium 866.23mg	36%
Total Carbohydrate 36g	12%
Dietary Fiber 3.41g	13%
Sugars 3.53g	
Protein 27.7g	55%

	Est. Percent of Calories from:
Fat	28%
Carbs	40%
Protein	30%

Turkey Stroganoff Casserole

Time: 45 mins
Servings: 6

Ingredients:
1 lb Turkey, Ground
5 cups (dry) Whole Wheat Wide Egg Noodles
2 1/2 cups (2 cans) Cream Of Mushroom Soup 98% Fat Free
1/2 cup Light Sour Cream
1/2 tsp Paprika
2 tbsp Minced Onions
2/3 cup Fat Free Mozzarella Shredded Cheese
3/4 tsp Kosher Salt
3/4 tsp Pure Ground Black Pepper

Directions:
Preheat oven to 425. Spray casserole dish. Cook noodles. Drain. Brown Turkey. Add in minced onions, paprika, soup, salt and pepper (and any other flavors to taste). Heat to a boil. Stir in sour cream. Heat through.
Pour noodles into dish, then top with meat mixture. Fold to mix. Top with cheese.
Cook in oven for about 10-12 mins until cheese is melted and bubbly.

Caesar Chicken & Roasted Potatoes Bake

Time: 45-50 mins
Servings: 4

Instructions:
1 1/6 lb Chicken Breast
(4 med/l g boneless,
skinless breasts)
1/4 cup Fat Free Caesar
Dressing
5 medium Russet
Potatoes
1 tbsp Extra Virgin
Olive Oil
2 tbsp grated Parmesan
Cheese
1/4 tsp Italian Seasoning
1/3 cup Fat Free Caesar
Dressing

NUTRITION FACTS	
Serving Size: 1/4 dish	
Amount per Serving	
Calories 340	Calories from Fat 64.5
	% Daily Value *
Total Fat 7.17g	11%
Saturated Fat 1.58g	7%
Cholesterol 78.36mg	26%
Sodium 840.56mg	35%
Total Carbohydrate 42.99g	14%
Dietary Fiber 3.75g	15%
Sugars 7.25g	
Protein 34.34g	68%
	Est. Percent of Calories from:
Fat	18%
Carbs	50%
Protein	40%

Directions:
Preheat oven to 425.
Trim any extra fat from chicken breasts. Spray casserole dish.
Place chicken in dish evenly and as far from each other as
possible. Sprinkle seasoning onto chicken. Use 1/4 cup of
dressing and lightly brush on tops of chicken breasts.
Cut potatoes into 1 inch cubes and place in large bowl. Top
with olive oil and remaining dressing (1/3 cup). Toss to coat
well. Pour potatoes and mixture over chicken breasts in dish,
and spread evenly. Sprinkle Parmesan cheese evenly over top.
Cover dish with aluminum foil.
Bake for about 30-40 mins. Check after about 20 mins, and stir
potatoes around to ensure even cooking. Remove foil about 10
mins before cooking time is up.

Muffaletta Stuffed Chicken

Time: 45 mins
Servings: 4

Ingredients:
20 oz Chicken Breast (4
med boneless, skinless)
2 oz Hot Muffaletta Mix
2 tsp Ground Coriander
Seed
1 cup Mexican Blend
Shredded Cheese

NUTRITION FACTS	
Serving Size. 1 stuffed breasts	
Amount per Serving	
Calories 207	Calories from Fat 99.9
	% Daily Value *
Total Fat 11.1g	17%
Saturated Fat 3.9g	19%
Cholesterol 83mg	27%
Sodium 414.8mg	17%
Total Carbohydrate 1g	0%
Dietary Fiber 0g	0%
Sugars 0.4g	
Protein 27.2g	54%
Est. Percent of Calories from:	
Fat	47%
Carbs	1%
Protein	52%

Directions:
Preheat oven to 375.
Spray cooking dish with
non-stick spray.
Spray long sheet of plastic wrap with non-stick spray, place one
chicken breast on top of wrap, then cover on top with same
sheet. Flatten with another pan, rolling pin, etc. Remove top
layer of wrap. Sprinkle with cheese, coriander seed, and onion
powder (and any other spices/ herbs you desire). Then put a
small dollop of muffaletta mix, then wrap breast around it into a
tube-shape. Place in pan. Repeat with each breast.
After breasts are in pan, sprinkle remaining cheese on top, and
cook for about 30-35 mins until done.

Scalloped Potatoes & Fish Bake

Time: 1 hr
Servings: 4

Ingredients:
4 Russet Potatoes, thinly
sliced
1 1/4 cups (1 can) 98% Fat
Free Cream Of Celery
Soup
4 Whiting Fillets
1 tbsp Kraft Mayo With
Olive Oil
2 tbsp Lemon Juice
1/3 cup Mild Shredded
Reduced Fat Cheddar
Cheese
1/2 medium Yellow
Onion, thinly sliced
1/2 cup Fat Free Skim Milk

NUTRITION FACTS	
Serving Size: 1/4 dish	
Amount per Serving	
Calories 295	Calories from Fat 50.0
	% Daily Value *
Total Fat 5.56g	8%
Saturated Fat 1.63g	8%
Cholesterol 53.75mg	17%
Sodium 641.85mg	26%
Total Carbohydrate 35.88g	11%
Dietary Fiber 3.93g	15%
Sugars 5.83g	
Protein 29.33g	58%
	Est. Percent of Calories from:
Fat	15%
Carbs	48%
Protein	39%

Directions:
Preheat Oven 425. Spray baking dish with non-stick spray.
Combine Cream of Celery Soup, mayonnaise, milk, and lemon
juice. Add any seasonings (salt, pepper, paprika, etc) as you wish
to taste. Coat the bottom of baking pan with 1/2 of the
mixture.
Place 1/2 of onion slices over mixture, then 1/2 of potatoes
over onions. Then lay fillets on top of potatoes. Sprinkle the
remaining onion evenly over the fillets, then layer the remaining
potato slices evenly over the top of the onion. Cover the top of
the potato slices with the remaining sauce mixture. Sprinkle the
shredded cheese evenly over the top. COVER the baking dish
with foil. Bake for 40-50 minutes. Remove foil and bake an
additional 10 minutes to brown top slightly.

Cajun Shrimp Luan

Time: 30 mins
Servings: 4

Ingredients:
9 oz Whole Wheat Thin
Spaghetti
1 tsp Chopped Garlic
14 oz (1 bag) Frozen
Small Cooked Shrimp
1 tbsp Extra Virgin
Olive Oil
2 tsp Seasoning
3 tbsp Salted Whipped
Butter

NUTRITION FACTS	
Serving Size: 1/4 batch	
Amount per Serving	
Calories 423	Calories from Fat 103.0
	% Daily Value *
Total Fat 11.44g	17%
Saturated Fat 3.13g	15%
Cholesterol 209.6mg	69%
Sodium 937.52mg	39%
Total Carbohydrate 46.38g	15%
Dietary Fiber 5.63g	22%
Sugars 2.25g	
Protein 32.38g	64%
Est. Percent of Calories from:	
Fat	23%
Carbs	43%
Protein	30%

Directions:
Cook pasta as directed on box.
Meanwhile, add all ingredients (keep shrimp frozen until adding) into pot and simmer covered (stirring occasionally) on med heat together. Drain cooked pasta. Pour shrimp mixture over pasta, stir/ toss several times until most of liquid is soaked up. Serve.

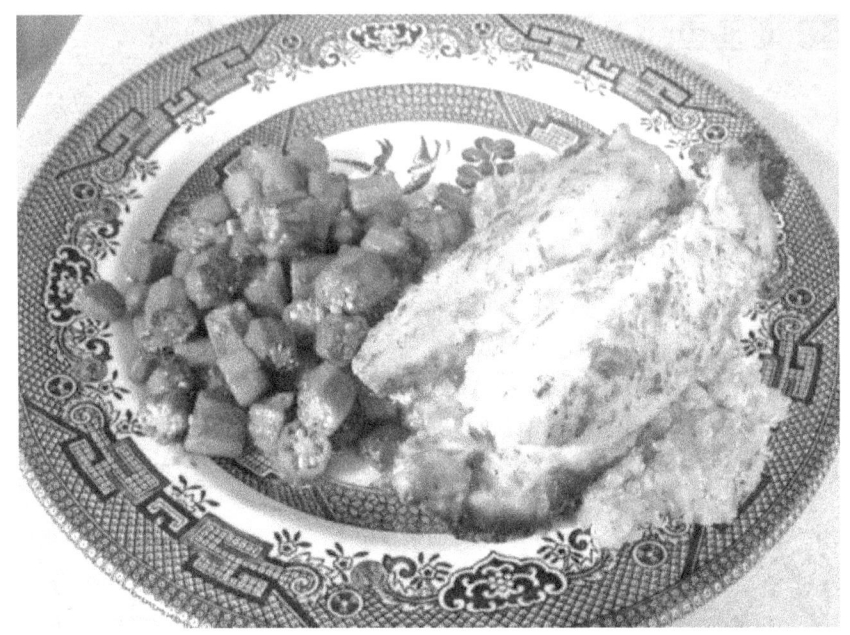

Orange Herb Chicken & Quinoa

NUTRITION FACTS	
Serving Size: 1 breast	
Amount per Serving	
Calories 329	Calories from Fat 47.0
	% Daily Value *
Total Fat 5.22g	8%
Saturated Fat 0.64g	3%
Cholesterol 81.25mg	27%
Sodium 948.94mg	39%
Total Carbohydrate 37.55g	12%
Dietary Fiber 4.91g	19%
Sugars 5.36g	
Protein 35.02g	70%

Orange Herb Chicken & Quinoa

Time: 45 minutes
Servings: 6 (1 breast & about ½ cup cooked quinoa each)

Ingredients:
30 oz boneless skinless chicken breasts (6 med)
1 tbsp Garlic Minced
2 tsp grated Orange Peel
1 1/2 tsp Kosher Salt
1 tsp Dried Thyme
1 tsp Dried Rosemary
1/2 tsp Ground Black Pepper
1 cup Light Orange Juice
3 tbsp Distilled White Vinegar
2 tbsp Worcestershire Sauce
1 1/2 cups (dry) plain Quinoa

Directions:
The night/ morning before cooking this meal: In large bowl,
combine orange peel & juice, garlic & herbs, salt & pepper,
Worcestershire sauce, and vinegar. Using a fork, stab chicken
breasts 4 times on each side. Place chicken in bowl with
mixture, and toss to coat well. Cover and refrigerate until ready
to cook.
Preheat/ clean grill. Begin to prepare quinoa as directed on
packaging, using about 2-3 tbsp less of water than called-for,
and replace with 2 tbsp orange herb mix.
Place chicken on prepared grill. Turn and baste with remaining
orange herb mix every 4-5 minutes. Grill for about 20-25
minutes until chicken is tender and thoroughly cooked.
Serve chicken over quinoa.

Corned-Beef Cabbage Rolls

Time: 75-80 mins
Servings: 8

Ingredients:
1 large head of cabbage
3 cups of diced,
cooked corned beef
(approx 16 oz.)
3 cups of diced,
cooked potatoes
(approx 3 md russet
potatoes)
1 tsp dried thyme
1 large egg white,
slightly beaten
1 cup of beef broth
2 tablespoons of
whipped butter
2 tablespoons of whole
wheat flour
1 cup of fat free skim
milk
1 cup of reduced fat shredded cheddar
salt and pepper to taste

NUTRITION FACTS	
Serving Size: 1 rolls	
Amount per Serving	
Calories 177	Calories from Fat 59.9
	% Daily Value *
Total Fat 6.66g	10%
Saturated Fat 3.13g	15%
Cholesterol 34.38mg	11%
Sodium 827.75mg	34%
Total Carbohydrate 16.48g	5%
Dietary Fiber 2.17g	8%
Sugars 3.53g	
Protein 13.09g	26%
Est. Percent of Calories from:	
Fat	31%
Carbs	37%
Protein	29%

Directions:
To begin, preheat your oven to 350°. Now take your cabbage and separate the leaves. Place the leaves in a large pot. Pour a small amount of water into the pot. Then, cover the pot and bring the water to a slight boil- to allow the leaves to steam slightly. Steam them until they are slightly wilted and flexible. Next, Add the corned beef to a large bowl. Then pour in the potatoes. Add the thyme. Sprinkle with salt. Add the pepper.

Corned-Beef Cabbage Rolls (cont'd)

Finally Add the egg. Now blend the mixture well.

Next take out a large baking dish and set the cabbage leaves inside. After, roll a portion of the mixture into a small ball that will fit into the cabbage leaf. Center the mixture in the middle of a cabbage leaf. Fold the sides of the cabbage around the corned beef. Now roll up leaf around the corned beef. Continue this process with the remaining ingredients and leaves. Before baking, pour the beef broth over the cabbage. Cover the baking dish with a lid or aluminum foil. Bake at 350° for 30 to 40 minutes.

Sauce: While the cabbage rolls are baking, prepare the sauce. Add 2 tablespoons of butter to a sauce pan and melt over medium heat. Add the flour. Now stir until the mixture is fully blended. Pour in the milk. Stir well. Keep simmering and stirring until the mixture thickens. Now sprinkle in the cheese. Keep cooking until the cheese is melted and the mixture is smooth. Next, add salt to taste. Then add pepper, to taste. Finally, Drizzle the cheese sauce over the cabbage rolls before serving.

Rosemary Roasted Chicken & Red Potatoes

Time: 1hr
Servings: 6

Ingredients:
4 Skinless Chicken
Thighs
3 Boneless, Skinless
Chicken Breasts (15
oz)
1 tbsp & 1 tsp Extra
Virgin Olive Oil
1 tsp Kosher Salt
1 1/2 lb red potato
2 tsp Paprika
1 1/2 tsp dried
Rosemary Leaves
1 tsp Minced Garlic
1/2 tsp Ground
Black Pepper

NUTRITION FACTS	
Serving Size: 1/6 batch	
Amount per Serving	
Calories 251	Calories from Fat 82.0
	% Daily Value *
Total Fat 9.11g	14%
Saturated Fat 2.06g	10%
Cholesterol 50mg	16%
Sodium 426.5mg	17%
Total Carbohydrate 20.09g	6%
Dietary Fiber 2.3g	9%
Sugars 2.3g	
Protein 25.39g	50%
Est. Percent of Calories from:	
Fat	32%
Carbs	31%
Protein	40%

Directions:
Preheat oven to 425.
Spray rack in roasting dish - OR - Line 15x10x1 baking pan
with foil and spray w/ non-stick spray. Cut potatoes into 1"
cubes.
Mix oil (use about 2 tbsp, but you'll only have about 1.3 tbsp on
the food after it drips off), spices, and salt in large bowl & whisk
well. Add chicken and potatoes and mix well to coat. Put
chicken and potatoes in single layer on pan.
Roast uncovered in oven for about 45 mins or until chicken is
cooked through and potatoes are tender, turning potatoes
occasionally.

Mouth-Watering Lemon Chicken & Rice

Time: 45 mins
Servings: 4

Ingredients:
20 oz Skinless,
Boneless Chicken
Breast (4 med breasts)
1 1/4 cups 98% Fat
Free Cream Of
Chicken (1 can)
2 tbsp Tap Water
2 tsp Parsley, Dried
2 tbsp Lemon Juice
1 tsp Paprika
1 cup Brown Rice

NUTRITION FACTS	
Serving Size 1/4 batch	
Amount per Serving	
Calories 366	Calories from Fat 67.8
	% Daily Value *
Total Fat 7.53g	11%
Saturated Fat 1.88g	9%
Cholesterol 68.75mg	22%
Sodium 669.92mg	27%
Total Carbohydrate 41.7g	13%
Dietary Fiber 2.91g	11%
Sugars 0.73g	
Protein 5.38g	10%
Est. Percent of Calories from:	
Fat	17%
Carbs	45%
Protein	5%

Directions:
Cook brown rice as directed and set aside. Meanwhile: Spray
nonstick skillet with cooking spray and heat over med-high heat
for 1 min. Add chicken and cook about 10 mins of until well
browned on both sides remove chicken from skillet.
Stir soup, water, parsley, lemon juice, and paprika in skillet and
heat to boil. Return chicken to skillet. Reduce heat to low.
Cover and cook about 5 mins or until chicken is cooked
through. Serve with/ over brown rice.

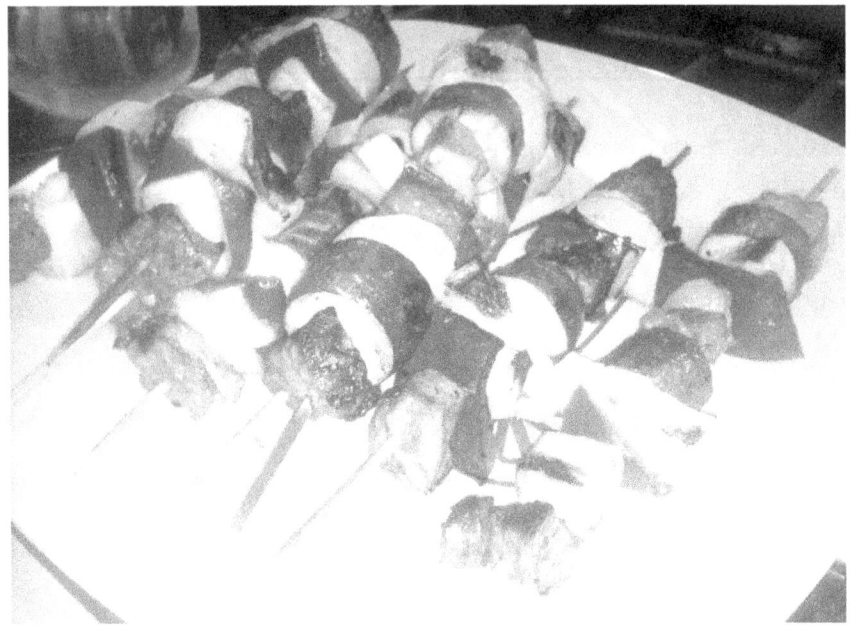

Greek Beef Kabobs & Couscous

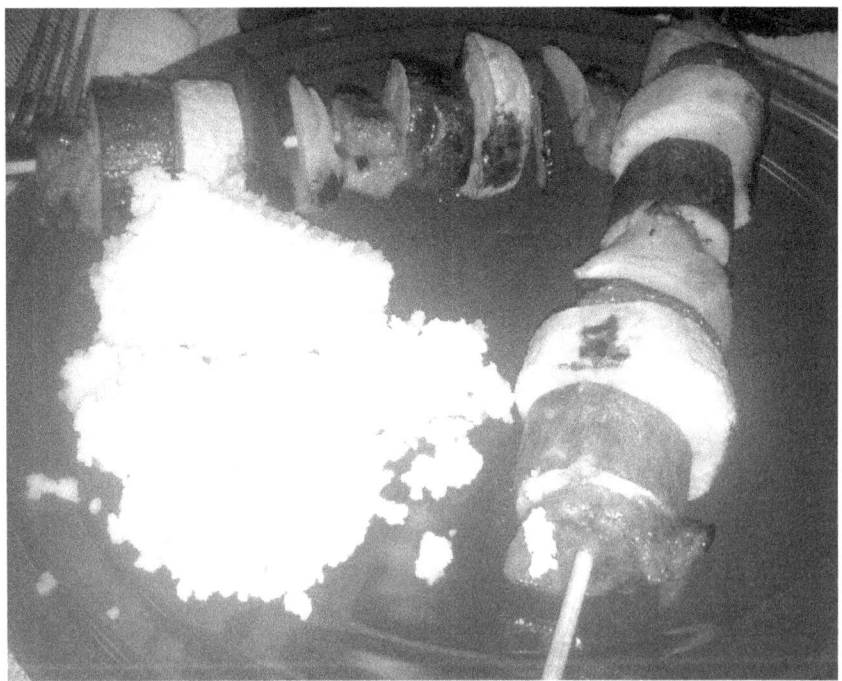

Greek Beef Kabobs & Couscous

Time: 30 mins (not including marinating time)
Servings: 6 (2 kabobs & ¾ cup couscous)

Ingredients:
18 oz Beef Sirloin Strip Steak, cut into 1" cubes
3 zucchinis, sliced ½" thick
3 medium Yellow Squashes, sliced ½" thick
3 Red Bell Peppers, cut into squares
2 medium Yellow Onions, cut into chunks
1/2 cup Light Greek Salad Dressing
1 1/2 cups (dry) Wheat Couscous

NUTRITION FACTS	
Serving Size: 2 kabobs	
Amount per Serving	
Calories 428	Calories from Fat 152.5
	% Daily Value *
Total Fat 16.94g	26%
Saturated Fat 5.78g	28%
Cholesterol 56.25mg	18%
Sodium 204.55mg	8%
Total Carbohydrate 43.47g	14%
Dietary Fiber 7.1g	28%
Sugars 11.05g	
Protein 24.87g	49%

Directions:
Combine meat, vegetables, and dressing into large plastic bag with zippered top. Marinate 4-6 hours in refrigerator.
Remove meat and vegetables from bag. Then stick meat and veggies onto 12 skewers (alternate meat, zucchini, squash, pepper, and onion, then repeat).
Prep Option 1: Pour remaining marinade into large skillet and bring to a boil. Boil skewers in skillet and baste with marinade 5-7 minutes or to desired doneness.
Prep Option 2: Grill kabobs and baste with remaining marinade as you grill.
Meanwhile, prepare couscous as directed on package (makes about 4.5 cups prepared). Serve kabobs over couscous.

Turkey Shepherd's Pie

Time: 45 mins
Servings: 6

Ingredients:
2 cups Instant Mashed
Potatoes
1 lb Turkey, Ground
1 3/4 cups (1 can) Sweet
Peas, Canned
1 3/4 cups (1 can) Sliced
Carrots
1 3/4 cups (1 can) Whole
Kernel Golden Corn
1/2 tsp Chicken Flavor
Instant Bouillion Granules
2 1/2 tbsp Minced Onions
2 tsp Garlic Powder
1 tsp Rubbed Sage
1 tsp Dried Basil Leaves
1/4 cup Reduced Fat Cream Cheese
1/2 cup Mild Shredded Reduced Fat Cheddar Cheese
1 tsp Worcestershire Sauce
2 tsp Coarse Kosher Salt
3/4 cup Fat Free Skim Milk
3 tbsp Light Margarine

NUTRITION FACTS	
Serving Size: 1/6 dish	
Amount per Serving	
Calories 380	Calories from Fat 103.1
	% Daily Value *
Total Fat 11.45g	17%
Saturated Fat 4.21g	21%
Cholesterol 64.91mg	21%
Sodium 1531.87mg	63%
Total Carbohydrate 36.3g	12%
Dietary Fiber 6.67g	26%
Sugars 10.58g	
Protein 24.3g	48%
Est. Percent of Calories from:	
Fat	26%
Carbs	38%
Protein	25%

Directions:
Preheat oven to 400. Make instant potatoes (6 servings) as
directed using 3 tbsp light margarine and 3/4 cup skim milk.
Meanwhile, add turkey, minced onions, and seasonings to large
pan to brown.

Turkey Shepherd's Pie (cont'd)

When almost browned, add vegetables, Worcestershire sauce, and broth (mix granules with about 1/2 cup of hot water). Turn to med/low heat and slowly warm.

In large bowl, add cream cheese. On top, add potatoes, and mix well. Add salt/ pepper to taste.

Spray dish. Add meat mixture. Spread potatoes on top. Sprinkle cheese evenly over top.

Bake at 400 for 20-30 mins (to desired color).

Cheesy Chicken, Broccoli, & Rice Casserole

Time: 60 mins
Servings: 6

Ingredients:
26 oz Boneless, Skinless Chicken Breast (4-5 med/lg breasts)
1 cup Brown Rice
1 1/4 cups (1 can) 98% Fat Free Cream of Broccoli Soup
1 (14 oz.) bag Frozen Broccoli Florets
1/2 cup Mild Shredded Reduced Fat Cheddar Cheese

NUTRITION FACTS	
Serving Size: 1/6 casserole	
Amount per Serving	
Calories 316	Calories from Fat 72.7
	% Daily Value *
Total Fat 8.08g	12%
Saturated Fat 2.5g	12%
Cholesterol 93.75mg	31%
Sodium 743.33mg	30%
Total Carbohydrate 31g	10%
Dietary Fiber 3.08g	12%
Sugars 1.92g	
Protein 29.33g	58%
Est. Percent of Calories from:	
Fat	21%
Carbs	39%
Protein	37%

Directions:
Par cook rice with 1 cup water instead of 2, then remove from heat when water is absorbed, then use in recipe:
Preheat oven to 450. Spray casserole dish with nonstick spray. Rough cut chicken breasts into large chunks. Stir rice, soup, and 1/2 cup of water and pour into dish. Sprinkle chicken chunks and broccoli florets evenly over rice mixture. Top with shredded cheese.
Bake approx 30-40 mins.

Classic Jambalaya

Time: 75 mins
Servings: 8

Ingredients:
1 3/4 cups Petite Diced
Tomatoes
3 1/4 cups Tomato
Puree
14 oz Minced Clams
14 oz Skinless Turkey
Smoked Sausage
1 1/4 cups Crab Meat -
Flake Style
15 oz (1 bag) frozen
small Shrimp
1 tsp Hot Sauce
1 medium yellow Onion
3 Large Celery Stalk
(11"-12" Long)
1 tbsp Chicken Flavor
Instant Bouillion Granules
1 large Green Bell Pepper
1 cup Brown Rice
1 tbsp Minced Garlic

NUTRITION FACTS	
Serving Size .2 cup	
Amount per Serving	
Calories 350	Calories from Fat 71.2
	% Daily Value *
Total Fat 7.91g	12%
Saturated Fat 2.19g	10%
Cholesterol 139.69mg	46%
Sodium 1645.61mg	68%
Total Carbohydrate 41.14g	13%
Dietary Fiber 4.16g	16%
Sugars 8.91g	
Protein 28.15g	56%
Est. Percent of Calories from:	
Fat	19%
Carbs	46%
Protein	32%

Directions:
Chop vegetables. Sweat onions. Add veggies and garlic into pot.
Chop sausage, add to pot. Add clams and tomatoes and puree
UNDRAINED. Add can & 1/2 of water with chicken granules.
Add rice. Simmer on medium until rice is done, then add
shrimp and crab. Add hot sauce and seasonings. Season with:
garlic powder, Cajun seasoning, pepper, crushed red pepper
flake, bay leaf (to taste).

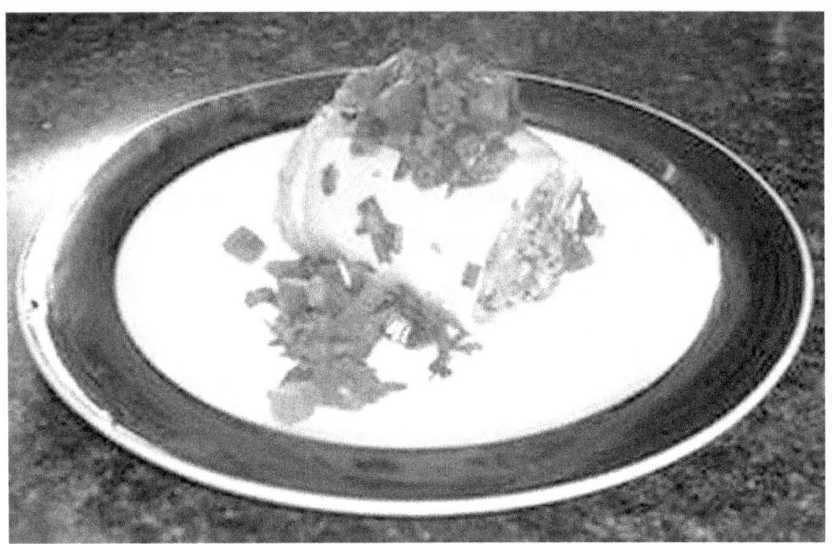

Italian Stuffed Chicken Breasts

NUTRITION FACTS

Serving Size: 1 stuffed breasts

Amount per Serving	
Calories 355	Calories from Fat 118.7

	% Daily Value *
Total Fat 13.19g	20%
Saturated Fat 3.63g	18%
Cholesterol 111.66mg	37%
Sodium 914.72mg	38%
Total Carbohydrate 23.13g	7%
Dietary Fiber 2.35g	9%
Sugars 3.05g	
Protein 35.1g	70%

Est. Percent of Calories from:	
Fat	33%
Carbs	26%
Protein	39%

Italian Stuffed Chicken Breasts

Time: 45 mins
Servings: 4

Ingredients:
20 oz Boneless, Skinless Chicken Breast (4 med breasts)
1 cup Plain Bread Crumbs
1 1/2 cups raw Spinach
1/2 Tomato
1/3 cup Shredded Part-Skim Mozarella
1/3 cup grated Parmesan Cheese
1 1/2 tbsp Italian Seasoning
1 tsp Garlic Powder
2 tbsp Mayonnaise With Olive Oil
1 tsp Extra Virgin Olive Oil

Directions:
Preheat oven to 400 degrees. Chop spinach and tomatoes and mix into bread crumbs. Add cheeses and stir well. Add Italian seasoning and garlic powder and stir well. Lastly, mix in mayo well and press down into bowl to ensure well absorption. Split stuffing mixture into 4 even portions.
Lay out each chicken breast on a large piece of plastic wrap (spray both sides of wrap with Pam for easier spreading), and pull wrap back over breast. Pound as flat as possible without tearing (about ¼" thick).
Spray a 8"x8" pan (glass is what I use) and set aside.
Take one portion of stuffing mix and make into a tight ball with your hands. Put at one end of flattened chicken breast and roll up - then place in pan. Do this for each breast. The breasts should be touching in pan to hold each other together. Bake for about 35 minutes.

Light & Delicious Chicken Tacos

Time: 20 mins
Servings: 4 (8 tacos total)

Ingredients:
1 lb Boneless, Skinless
Chicken Breasts
4 tbsp Light Sour
Cream
1 tbsp Taco Seasoning
Mix/ Powder
8 Life Balance Flour
Tortilla - Medium
8 tbsp Medium Salsa
1 tbsp Salted
Whipped Butter
3/4 cup Reduced Fat
Shredded Cheddar
Cheese

NUTRITION FACTS	
Serving Size: 2 tacos	
Amount per Serving	
Calories 432	Calories from Fat 123.6
	% Daily Value *
Total Fat 13.73g	21%
Saturated Fat 6.38g	31%
Cholesterol 85.81mg	28%
Sodium 1297.13mg	54%
Total Carbohydrate 45.5g	15%
Dietary Fiber 8g	32%
Sugars 5.38g	
Protein 36.38g	72%
Est. Percent of Calories from:	
Fat	23%
Carbs	42%
Protein	33%

Directions:
Cut chicken into small
chunks. Cook in skillet over med-high heat with taco seasoning,
butter, and 1/3 cup water. Once cooked, assemble tacos in flour
tortillas with toppings and veggies (i.e. lettuce, tomato, sliced
bell peppers).

Sausage & Rigatoni w/ Caramelized Onions & Tomato Sauce

Time: 35 mins
Servings: 6 (about 2 oz. dry pasta, 1/6 sausage mix each)

Ingredients:
1 cup Olive Oil & Garlic Tomato Sauce
5 link Mild Italian Sausage
1 medium Red Onion
2 tsp Minced Garlic
1/2 tbsp Extra Virgin Olive Oil
12 oz Whole Wheat Veggie Rigatoni

NUTRITION FACTS	
Serving Size: 1/6 batch	
Amount per Serving	
Calories 485	Calories from Fat 193.1
	% Daily Value *
Total Fat 21.46g	33%
Saturated Fat 7.67g	38%
Cholesterol 50mg	16%
Sodium 774.17mg	32%
Total Carbohydrate 50.83g	16%
Dietary Fiber 7.5g	30%
Sugars 6.67g	
Protein 22.67g	45%
Est. Percent of Calories from:	
Fat	41%
Carbs	41%
Protein	18%

Directions:
Begin cooking pasta as directed on box.
Meanwhile, cut onion in half and very thinly slice. Heat olive oil over med-med/high heat in a large skillet, then add onion. Cook until brown and soft.
Meanwhile, cut up sausages into small bits. Once onion is cooked, add sausage bits and minced garlic. Cook over medium - med/high heat until sausage is fully cooked. Reduce heat to low, cover and let simmer for 3-5 mins, stirring occasionally.
Stir in tomato sauce, cover again and continue simmering until heated through. Serve over rigatoni.

Cream of Mushroom Chicken & Rice Casserole

Time: 60-70 mins
Servings: 6

Ingredients:
32 oz Boneless
Skinless Chicken
Breast (6 med
breasts)
2 1/2 cups (2 cans)
98% Fat Free Cream
of Mushroom Soup
1 1/2 cups Brown
Rice
2 1/2 cups water
1 tbsp Italian
Seasoning
1 tsp Coarse Kosher
Salt
1 tsp Pure Ground
Black Pepper

NUTRITION FACTS

Serving Size: 1 breasts and rice

Amount per Serving	
Calories 367	Calories from Fat 62.3

	% Daily Value *
Total Fat 6.92g	10%
Saturated Fat 1.08g	5%
Cholesterol 90.83mg	30%
Sodium 964.5mg	40%
Total Carbohydrate 42.5g	14%
Dietary Fiber 2.83g	11%
Sugars 0g	
Protein 35.5g	71%

Est. Percent of Calories from:	
Fat	16%
Carbs	46%
Protein	38%

Directions:
Preheat oven to 425 F. Grease/ spray dish.
In large bowl, whisk 2 cans of soup, 2 cans of water, 1.5 cups of rice, Italian seasoning, salt, and pepper.
Pour mix into dish and evenly spread rice. Evenly place chicken breasts on top.
After 40 mins, stir around rice then continue cooking. After another 20 mins, check to make sure rice is fully cooked. If not, stir and continue to cook in 10 minute increments until tender. If it is, fluff rice with a fork then serve.

Cajun Chicken & Dumplings

Time: 45 mins
Servings: 8

Ingredients:
2 1/2 lb Boneless
Skinless Chicken Breasts
3 cups low cholesterol/
low fat biscuit mix
1 1/2 cups Fat Free Skim
Milk
18 cups Water
1 tbsp Cajun Seasoning
2 tbsp Chicken Flavor
Instant Bouillon Granules
3/4 tbsp Garlic Powder

NUTRITION FACTS	
Serving Size 3 cup	
Amount per Serving	
Calories 316	Calories from Fat 53.5
	% Daily Value *
Total Fat 5.94g	9%
Saturated Fat 0.63g	3%
Cholesterol 82.19mg	27%
Sodium 1754.06mg	73%
Total Carbohydrate 33.56g	11%
Dietary Fiber 1.13g	4%
Sugars 5.06g	
Protein 33.81g	67%
Est. Percent of Calories from:	
Fat	16%
Carbs	42%
Protein	42%

Directions:
In a big pot, boil chicken in about 18 cups of water with salt & pepper (to taste), granules, and Tony's seasoning for added flavor. Once cooked (about 25-35 mins), remove chicken (Do NOT drain water!) and shred with forks.
Meanwhile, mix up biscuit mix with milk to make lumpy batter and let rest to rise.
Put chicken back in broth and bring back to a boil.
Reduce to medium heat. Drop large tablespoonfuls of batter into boiling water to create "dumplings".
Once done dropping dumplings, let them expand/ cook for about 5 mins in the covered pot on low heat, stirring gently as you go to mix up dumplings. Then, turn off heat. The longer you let it sit, the thicker the broth will become.

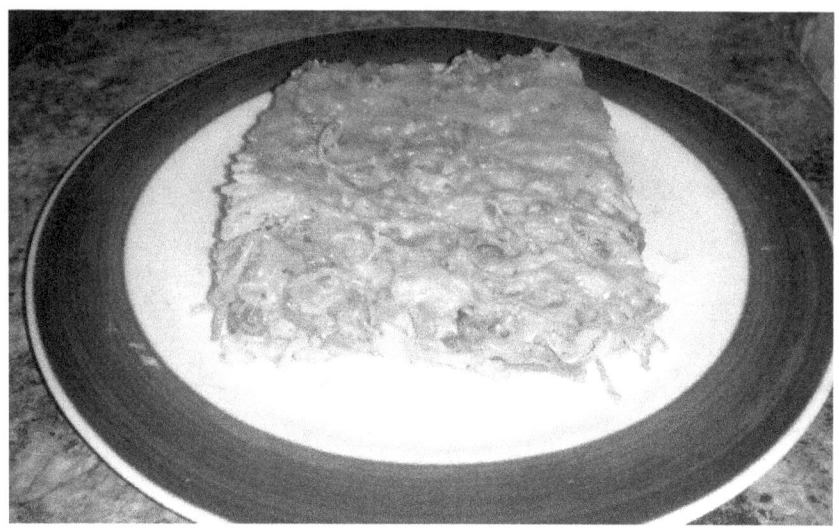

<u>Cheesy Tuna Noodle Casserole</u>

NUTRITION FACTS

Serving Size: 1/8 casserole

Amount per Serving

Calories 336	Calories from Fat 54.3

	% Daily Value *
Total Fat 6.03g	9%
Saturated Fat 2.44g	12%
Cholesterol 24.69mg	8%
Sodium 647.44mg	26%
Total Carbohydrate 50.53g	16%
Dietary Fiber 6.88g	27%
Sugars 6.78g	
Protein 17.84g	35%

Est. Percent of Calories from:	
Fat	15%
Carbs	60%
Protein	21%

Cheesy Tuna Noodle Casserole

Time: 40 mins
Servings: 6

Ingredients:
12 oz (dry) Whole Wheat Thin Spaghetti
8 oz (2 cans) Chunk Light Tuna in Water (drained)
3 1/3 cups (1 16oz frozen bag) Mixed Vegetables
3 tbsp Whole Wheat Flour
1 1/2 cups Unsweetened Vanilla Almond Milk
3 tbsp Salted Whipped Butter
1 cup Mild Shredded Reduced Fat Cheddar Cheese
1 tbsp All Purpose Greek Seasoning

Directions:
Preheat oven to 375. Spray a (11x13) 4 quart casserole dish with cooking spray.
In a large pot of salted water, boil noodles until al dente. Drain well, then return to pot.
In a medium saucepan on low heat, combine flour, butter, and seasoning. Stir until butter is melted and ingredients are combined evenly.
Increase heat to med heat and add milk, and whisk until the sauce thickens (usually it is at the proper consistency by the time it begins to boil). Add 2/3 cup of cheese to mixture, and whisk until cheese is melted and mixture is well blended. Fold in tuna and vegetables, then pour over noodles and toss/mix well. Spread evenly in prepared dish. Sprinkle remaining 1/3 cup cheese over the top. Bake in preheated oven for 10-15 minutes or until cheese is melted and bubbly.

Teriyaki Chicken Lettuce Wraps w/ Rice & Broccoli

Time: 45 mins
Servings: 4 (2 wraps, 1/2 cup cooked rice, & 1.25 cup broccoli each)

Ingredients:
18 oz Boneless Skinless Chicken Breast
2 cups Bibb Lettuce (8 large leafs)
2 tbsp Salted Whipped Butter
1 tbsp 100% Pure Cornstarch
1 large Egg White
1 tbsp Chinese Rice Wine Vinegar
1 tbsp Minced Onion
2 tsp Minced Garlic
2/3 cup Low Sodium Teriyaki Sauce
2 tsp Ground Mustard
3 tsp Ground Ginger
5 cups frozen Broccoli Florets
1 cup Brown Rice

NUTRITION FACTS	
Serving Size: 2 wraps	
Amount per Serving	
Calories 415	Calories from Fat 69.8
	% Daily Value *
Total Fat 7.76g	11%
Saturated Fat 2.31g	11%
Cholesterol 80.63mg	26%
Sodium 1101.96mg	45%
Total Carbohydrate 51.41g	17%
Dietary Fiber 4.5g	18%
Sugars 9.31g	
Protein 33.48g	66%
Est. Percent of Calories from:	
Fat	15%
Carbs	49%
Protein	32%

Directions:
Cook rice as directed. Gently remove 8 large leaves of lettuce for wraps.
Cut chicken into 1" chunks. Whisk cornstarch, egg white, and rice wine vinegar in mixing bowl, then toss chicken chunks to coat well. Heat butter in large skillet on med/high heat, and when hot, add chicken to cook.

Teriyaki Chicken Lettuce Wraps w/ Rice & Broccoli (cont'd)

Stir and flip pieces only a couple times each, being careful not to strip the coating. When chicken is thoroughly cooked (about 15-20 mins), remove from skillet and place on paper towels to dry.

Add Teriyaki sauce, ginger, minced onions, minced garlic, and mustard to skillet on med/high heat, stirring well to blend. When hot, add broccoli. Put on lid and simmer 10-15 mins until tender, stirring often. Remove broccoli from sauce, but SAVE sauce and set to the side.

Spread out lettuce leaf, portion out chicken on one end of leaf, and drizzle sauce over chicken, then wrap. Repeat for all 8 leaves.

Serve with rice and broccoli on the side.

Meaty, Cheesy, Veggie Casserole with a Kick!

Time: 35 mins
Servings: 6 (about 2 cups each)

Ingredients:
1 lb Turkey, Ground
3 cups (1 box)
Reduced fat shells and
cheese
4 cups Frozen Mixed
Vegetables
2/3 cup Mild
Shredded Reduced Fat
Cheddar Cheese
1/3 cup Light Sour
Cream
2 tsp Cajun Seasoning

NUTRITION FACTS

Serving Size: 2 cup

Amount per Serving	
Calories 386	Calories from Fat 96.2

	% Daily Value *
Total Fat 10.69g	16%
Saturated Fat 4.67g	23%
Cholesterol 71.94mg	23%
Sodium 1067.21mg	44%
Total Carbohydrate 41.89g	13%
Dietary Fiber 3g	12%
Sugars 8.39g	
Protein 27.55g	55%

Est. Percent of Calories from:	
Fat	24%
Carbs	43%
Protein	28%

Directions:
Preheat oven to 400.
Spray casserole dish.
Brown Turkey and
cook shells.
Prepare shells and cheese, then fold in sour cream, seasoning,
and browned turkey. Then fold in veggies. Pour into casserole
dish and cover evenly with shredded cheese.
Bake for 12-15 mins at 400.

Easy Pork Tenderloin & Apple Waldorf

Time: 1 hour (not including marinating time)
Servings: 6

Ingredients:
2 pork tenderloins (about 1.5 lbs total)
2/3 cup Apple Jelly
1/4 cup Lemon Juice
1/4 cup Light Soy Sauce
1/4 cup Unsweetened applesauce
1 tbsp Vegetable Oil
1 tbsp Ground Ginger
1 Red Delicious Apple, chopped
2 slices light wheat bread
– chopped/crumbled for bread crumbs (about 1 cup)
1/4 cup Chopped Pecans

NUTRITION FACTS	
Serving Size 1/3 stuffed tenderloins	
Amount per Serving	
Calories 311	Calories from Fat 78.0
	% Daily Value *
Total Fat 8.67g	13%
Saturated Fat 3g	15%
Cholesterol 0mg	0%
Sodium 363.2mg	15%
Total Carbohydrate 33.04g	11%
Dietary Fiber 1.83g	7%
Sugars 25.71g	
Protein 25.33g	50%

Directions:
Partially slice tenderloins length-wise (do NOT cut all the way through) and place in baking dish.

In small sauce pan, combine jelly, lemon juice, soy sauce, ginger, applesauce, and oil. Cook and stir until jelly is melted. Reserve about 3 tbsp of the mixture and set aside. Pour remaining jelly mix over tenderloins. Cover and refrigerate 4-6 hours or overnight.

When ready to cook: Preheat oven to 375 F. Combine bread crumbs, chopped apple, nuts, an reserved jelly mixture. Spread slits in meat open wide (being careful not to rip sides) and evenly fill with bread crumb stuffing.

Bake in oven uncovered for 30 minutes. Remove briefly and cover with aluminum foil and bake an additional 10 minutes (or until internal temperature of pork reaches 160F).

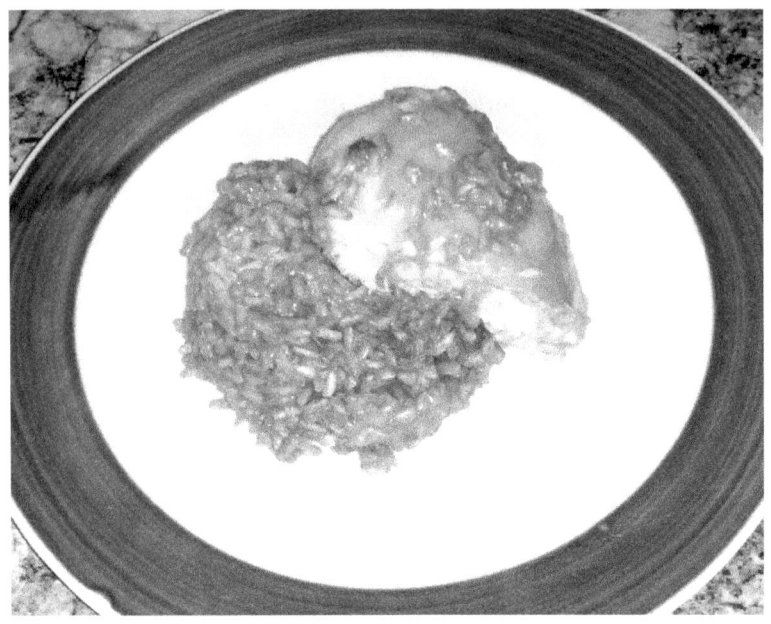

Fiesta Chicken Skillet

NUTRITION FACTS	
Serving Size: 1/5 skillet	
Amount per Serving	
Calories 378	Calories from Fat 73.4
	% Daily Value *
Total Fat 8.16g	12%
Saturated Fat 2.39g	11%
Cholesterol 85.5mg	28%
Sodium 728.72mg	30%
Total Carbohydrate 42.56g	14%
Dietary Fiber 2.66g	10%
Sugars 1.48g	
Protein 34.42g	68%
	Est. Percent of Calories from:
Fat	10%
Carbs	45%
Protein	36%

Fiesta Chicken Skillet

Time: 75 mins
Servings: 5

Ingredients:
24 oz Boneless, Skinless Chicken Breast
1/2 tbsp Extra Virgin Olive Oil
1 3/4 cups Condensed Tomato Soup
2 cups water
1 cup Brown Rice
2 tsp Chili Powder
1/2 cup Mild Shredded Reduced Fat Cheddar Cheese
1/2 tbsp Salted Whipped Butter

Directions:
Parcook rice first (as directed on packaging) with only 1 cup water, and remove from heat after water is absorbed. In large skillet, heat oil and butter over med-high heat and cook chicken until brown on both sides. Then remove chicken from skillet and set aside.
Bring soup, remaining water, and chili powder to a boil in skillet. Add in rice and stir well. Cover and reduce heat to med-low. Simmer for about 15-20 mins stirring occasionally. Stir rice mix, then add chicken on top of rice mixture. Top chicken with cheese.
Cover and simmer an additional 15-20 mins until rice is tender and chicken completely cooked. Stir rice before serving.

Bayou Pork Rollups

Time: 50 mins
Servings: 6 (1 serving = 2 rollup slices &
about 1 cup prepared rice)

Ingredients:
2 pork tenderloins
(3/4 lb each)
1/2 tbsp Extra Virgin
Olive Oil
1 red bell pepper,
chopped
1/2 medium red
onion, chopped
2 tsp Minced Garlic
1 tbsp Cajun
Seasoning
1 tbsp Fennel Seed,
crushed
2 tbsp Lemon Juice
2 tsp Ground Black
Pepper
2 tbsp Diced Green Chiles
1 1/2 cups (dry) Brown Rice

NUTRITION FACTS	
Serving Size: 2 slices rollups	
Amount per Serving	
Calories 380	Calories from Fat 74.6
	% Daily Value *
Total Fat 8.29g	12%
Saturated Fat 2.06g	10%
Cholesterol 88mg	29%
Sodium 133.67mg	5%
Total Carbohydrate 38.05g	12%
Dietary Fiber 2.96g	11%
Sugars 1.39g	
Protein 36.34g	72%

Directions:
Preheat oven to 325F. Spray shallow baking pan with nonstick
spray.
Going lengthwise down the center, cut tenderloins almost to
bottom, being careful not cutting all the way through. Open loin
from cut so it lays flat and cover with plastic wrap. Using a
mallet, working from the center of the loins to the edges, gently
flatten meat to about 1/4" thick them remove plastic wrap. Do
this for both loins.

Bayou Pork Rollups (cont'd)

Heat oil in large skillet to med-high heat. Add pepper, onion, chiles, onion, garlic, and cajun seasoning. Cook and stir for about 5 minutes or until vegetables are softened. Meanwhile, start cooking rice as directed on packaging (it should be finishing cooking around the same time as the rollups). Evenly spread veggie mixture over flattened tenderloins to within 1" of edges. Starting with the shorter sides, start carefully rolling, tucking sides as needed as you go so as not to spill any of the stuffing. Secure edges with toothpicks or tie rolls with cooking string. Place each roll, seam side down, in prepped baking dish. Mix crushed fennel seed, lemon juice, and pepper in small bowl. Brush each roll evenly with this mixture. Bake for about 25 minutes. Briefly pull out rolls and brush again with juice mix. Continue cooking for an additional 20 minutes or until pork is done (internal temperature reaches 155F). Remove from oven and let stand for 5 minutes. Remove toothpicks or string. Cut each roll into 6 slices. Serve with brown rice.

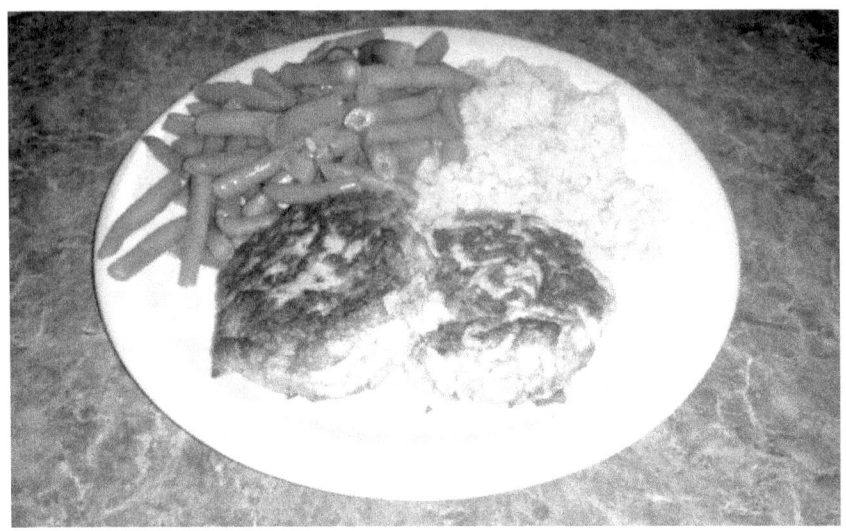

Spicy Cajun Crab Cakes

NUTRITION FACTS

Serving Size: 2 cakes

Amount per Serving

Calories 312	Calories from Fat 137.7

	% Daily Value *
Total Fat 15.3g	23%
Saturated Fat 1.75g	8%
Cholesterol 15.5mg	5%
Sodium 2227.5mg	92%
Total Carbohydrate 34.18g	11%
Dietary Fiber 0g	0%
Sugars 7.45g	
Protein 8.06g	16%

Spicy Cajun Crab Cakes

Time: 35 mins
Servings: 4 (Makes 8 cakes – 2 cakes per person)

Ingredients:
1 lb Crab Flavored Seafood
2 large Egg White
25 reduced fat round crackers, crumbled
1/2 cup Kraft Mayo With Olive Oil
1 tbsp Lemon Juice
2 tbsp Heinz Dill Relish
2 tbsp Salted Whipped Butter
1 tbsp Tony Cachere's Cajun Seasoning

Directions:
Mix mayo, egg whites, relish, seasoning, and lime juice in medium bowl. Add crushed crackers, and mix well. Then mix in flaked crab meat. Separate into 4 equal portions, then firmly shape into 8 even patties.
Heat butter in large skillet on med/high heat until butter is melted and hot. Add patties; cook about 5 min. on each side or until firm and golden brown on both sides. Place on paper towel and blot excess oil before serving.

BBQ Country Meatloaf & Mashed Potatoes

Time: 1 hour
Servings: 8 (1 serving = 1/8th loaf & mashed potatoes)

Ingredients:
1 lb Ground Venison
1 lb Ground Turkey
1 cup Plain Quick
Oatmeal
1 tbsp Ground Black
Pepper
2 large Egg Whites
¼ cup Sweet'n Spicy
BBQ Sauce
7 Idaho Potatoes,
peeled & cubed
¾ cup Unsweetened
Vanilla Almond Milk
1 1/2 tbsp Whipped
Butter
3/4 tsp Kosher Salt
1 1/2 tsp Ground Black Pepper
3 tbsp Sweet'n Spicy BBQ Sauce

NUTRITION FACTS	
Serving Size: 1/8 loaf	
Amount per Serving	
Calories 332	Calories from Fat 92.8
	% Daily Value *
Total Fat 10.31g	15%
Saturated Fat 1.78g	8%
Cholesterol 96.81mg	32%
Sodium 372.63mg	15%
Total Carbohydrate 30.12g	10%
Dietary Fiber 3.72g	14%
Sugars 5.56g	
Protein 28.87g	57%

Directions:
Preheat oven to 400F. Place parchment paper on cookie sheet
and lightly spray with nonstick spray.
Blend both meats, oatmeal, 1/4 cup BBQ sauce, egg whites, and
1 tbsp pepper by hand, tossing and folding meat over
ingredients, being careful not to over-mix.
Form meat mixture into loaf-shape on cookie sheet/ parchment
paper. Drizzle last 3 tbsp of BBQ sauce over loaf in a zig-zag
motion.
Bake in oven for 50-60 minutes until thoroughly cooked and
lightly browned on the outside.

BBQ Country Meatloaf & Mashed Potatoes (cont'd)

Meanwhile, put potato cubes in pot and cover with water. Bring to a boil and boil for about 15-20 minutes until tender. Drain. Add butter, almond milk, salt and pepper to potatoes. Mash well by hand or with hand mixer.

Slice loaf into 8 servings and serve with potatoes and green veggie of your choice.

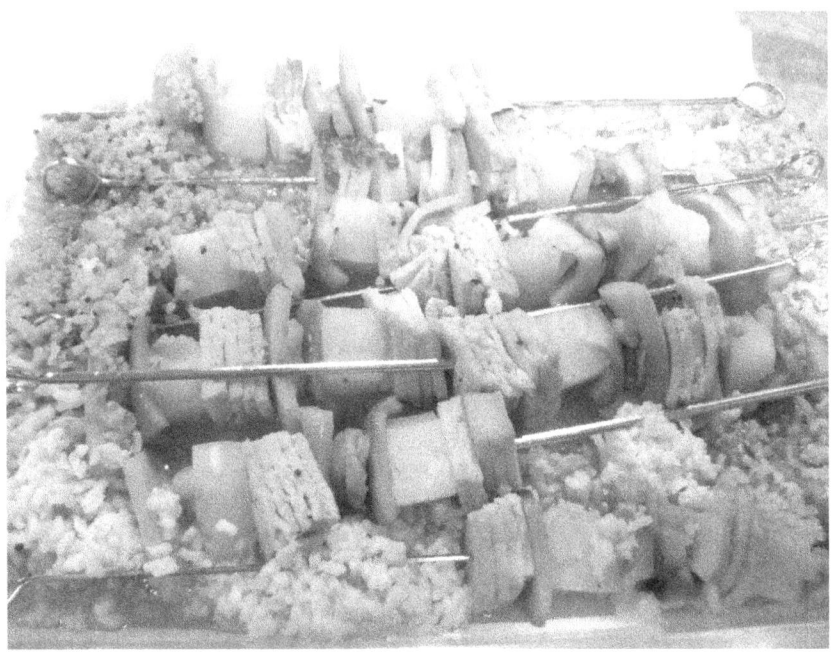

<u>Tangy Hawaiian Ham Skewers & Rice</u>

NUTRITION FACTS

Serving Size: 2 skewers

Amount per Serving

Calories 416	Calories from Fat 114.4

	% Daily Value *
Total Fat 12.71g	19%
Saturated Fat 3.04g	15%
Cholesterol 60mg	20%
Sodium 898.6mg	37%
Total Carbohydrate 58.6g	19%
Dietary Fiber 5.09g	20%
Sugars 18.23g	
Protein 19.27g	38%

Tangy Hawaiian Ham Skewers & Rice

Time: 45 mins
Servings: 4 (8 skewers & 3 cups rice prepared)

Ingredients:
12 oz Chopped Ham, cut into one-inch cubes
1 ¾ cup (1 can) no sugar added pineapple chunks
1 large Green Bell Pepper, cut into one-inch cubes
1 red bell pepper, cut into one-inch cubes
1 yellow bell pepper, cut into one-inch cubes
2 cups Button Mushrooms, halved
3 tbsp Light Raspberry Walnut Vinaigrette
1 cup (dry) Brown Rice

Directions:
Preheat oven to 350. Start cooking rice as directed on package. Let rice cook for about 30 minutes.
Lightly spray skewers and large baking dish with non-stick spray. Drain pineapple chunks and reserve juice from can. Skewer ham, pineapple chunks, peppers, and mushrooms by alternating onto wood or metal skewers. Place skewers into baking dish. Mix pineapple juice and dressing. Evenly brush all skewers with juice mix. Bake for about 8 minutes, then rotate all skewers and brush all ingredients well again with mix. Continue baking for about 8-10 minutes until heated through. Lightly brush one last time with mix immediately after removing from oven. Serve skewers over rice. (1 serving = 2 skewers and ½ cup cooked rice).

Chicken Curry & Couscous

Time: 30 mins
Servings: 6 (1 serving = 1/6th or about 2/3 cup skillet & about ¾ cup prepared couscous)

Ingredients:
24 oz Boneless, Skinless, Chicken Breast, cut into ½" cubes
1 medium Yellow Onion, chopped
1 1/2 medium Red Delicious Apples, chopped
1 medium Tomato, chopped
1 cup water
1/3 cup California Golden Raisins
3 tbsp Curry Powder
1 1/2 tsp Sodium Free Chicken Bouillon
1 tsp Minced Garlic
1 1/2 cups Wheat Couscous
2 tbsp Chopped Peanuts
2 tsp Extra Virgin Olive Oil

NUTRITION FACTS	
Serving Size: 1/6 skillet	
Amount per Serving	
Calories 361	Calories from Fat 77.4
	% Daily Value *
Total Fat 8.6g	13%
Saturated Fat 1.22g	6%
Cholesterol 50mg	16%
Sodium 254.39mg	10%
Total Carbohydrate 43.82g	14%
Dietary Fiber 4.36g	17%
Sugars 13.44g	
Protein 26.81g	53%

Directions:
Heat oil in large skillet to med-high heat. Add chicken and onion to skillet. Cook, stirring occasionally, until chicken is browned and onion is tender (about 10 minutes).
Meanwhile, begin cooking couscous as directed on package.
Then stir in apples, tomatoes, water, raisins, curry powder, bouillon granules, and minced garlic to skillet and mix well.
Reduce heat to low and cover and cook for about 10 minutes, stirring occasionally, until desired consistency.
Serve chicken mixture (about 2/3 cup) over couscous (3/4 cup prepared per serving), and sprinkle chopped peanuts on top.

Lean Sloppy Joes

Time: 30 minutes
Servings: 6

Ingredients:
1 lb lean ground turkey
1/2 medium Yellow Onions, chopped
1/2 large Green Bell Pepper, chopped
1/2 cup tomato ketchup
1/2 cup water
1 1/2 tsp Chili Powder
1/2 tsp Coarse Kosher Salt
1/4 tsp Ground Black Pepper
1 tsp Sriracha HOT Chili Sauce
6 Light Wheat Hamburger Buns

NUTRITION FACTS	
Serving Size: 1 sloppy joe	
Amount per Serving	
Calories 215	Calories from Fat 63.3
	% Daily Value *
Total Fat 7.03g	10%
Saturated Fat 1.68g	8%
Cholesterol 60mg	20%
Sodium 673.66mg	28%
Total Carbohydrate 27.05g	9%
Dietary Fiber 7.57g	30%
Sugars 8.58g	
Protein 18.53g	37%

Directions:
Spray large skillet with non stick spray, and heat over med-high heat. Add chopped onions, and bell peppers to skillet. Cook and stir until softened. Add turkey, stir and cook until browned. Drain well.
Return meat & veggie mix to skillet. Stir in ketchup, sriracha chili sauce, chili powder, salt, pepper, and water. Reduce heat to low. Cook about 15 minutes until thickened.
Evenly distribute onto buns to make sandwiches.

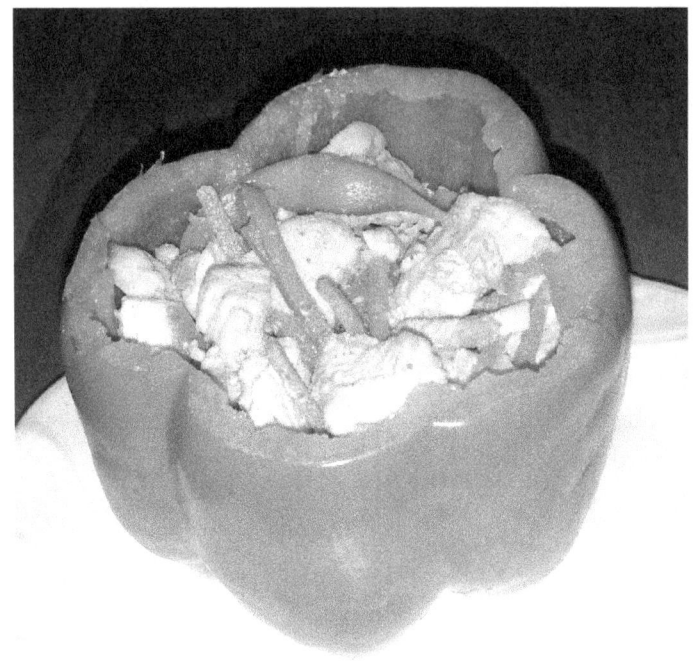

Teriyaki Chicken Peppers

NUTRITION FACTS

Serving Size: 1 stuffed peppers

Amount per Serving

Calories 295	Calories from Fat 34.5

	% Daily Value *
Total Fat 3.83g	5%
Saturated Fat 0.6g	3%
Cholesterol 65mg	21%
Sodium 784mg	32%
Total Carbohydrate 38.57g	12%
Dietary Fiber 4.92g	19%
Sugars 10.04g	
Protein 28.88g	57%

Teriyaki Chicken Peppers

Time: 1 hour 15 minutes
Servings: 6

Ingredients:
1 1/2 lb boneless, skinless Chicken Breast
6 large Green Bell Peppers
1 carrot, julienned (or cut into small thin strips)
1/3 cup Teriyaki Sauce Original
1 tsp Ground Ginger
1 cup Snow Pea Pods
1 cup (dry) Brown Rice
2 tbsp Low Sodium Soy Sauce

Directions:
Prepare rice as directed on packaging & preheat oven to 400F. Meanwhile, cut the very tops off of peppers, and remove seeds and scrape interior white stalks as much as possible (being careful not to puncture peppers). Trim excess fat off chicken, then cut up into small bits (no larger than 1/2"). When there is only 10-15 minutes left on the rice, heat large skillet to med-high heat and add teriyaki and soy sauces, and ginger; bring to a simmer. Then add chicken, carrots, and pea pods to skillet. Simmer and stir occasionally for 5-10 minutes.
Meanwhile, loosely cover baking dish with aluminum foil and spray lightly with non-stick spray. Place peppers on aluminum foil about 2" away from eachother, then crumple aluminum foil around and between the peppers to help them stand firmly.
For each pepper, pack about 1/3 prepared rice. Then evenly distribute the chicken and vegetable mixture into each pepper (leaving the sauce in the skillet). Then take about 1 tbsp of the remaining sauce and pour over the top of each pepper. Cover baking dish with foil.
Carefully place baking dish in oven and bake about 20 minutes until peppers are tender and chicken fully cooked.

Light & Easy Chicken Cordon Bleu

Time: 45 minutes
Servings: 6

Ingredients:
1.5 lb boneless skinless
chicken breasts (6 med)
1 tbsp Dijon mustard
1 tsp dried Thyme
1 tsp dried oregano
6 slices Lean Honey
Ham (deli ham)
3 Light Swiss Deli
Slices
1/4 cup Italian
Seasoned Bread Crumbs
2 tbsp Light Grated Parmesan

NUTRITION FACTS	
Serving Size: 1 rolled breast	
Amount per Serving	
Calories 197	Calories from Fat 53.6
	% Daily Value *
Total Fat 5.95g	9%
Saturated Fat 1.5g	7%
Cholesterol 67.08mg	22%
Sodium 714.39mg	29%
Total Carbohydrate 4.14g	1%
Dietary Fiber 0.36g	1%
Sugars 0.68g	
Protein 29.29g	58%

Directions:
Preheat oven to 400F. Spray large cut of plastic wrap with
nonstick spray. Combine breadcrumbs and parmesan cheese in
shallow dish. Spray baking dish with nonstick spray.
For each breast: Place on warp and pull wrap over to cover top
of breast. Pound evenly to about 1/4" thickness. Evenly spread
mustard down center. Sprinkle evenly with thyme and oregano.
Top with 1 slice of ham and 1/2 slice of cheese. Starting at
most narrow end, carefully roll up, being careful to tuck in sides
of ham and chicken to seal as you go. Secure with toothpicks as
needed. Breast should have some remaining non-stick spray on
it, but if needed, lightly brush with water. Gently roll in
breadcrumb mix. Place in baking dish. Repeat for each breast.
Bake for 10 minutes at 400. Then reduce oven temperature to
350F and continue baking for 20-25 minutes until chicken is
thoroughly cooked. Remove toothpicks before serving.

Chicken & Spinach Casserole

Time: 45 minutes
Servings: 6

Ingredients:
1.5 lb boneless skinless chicken breasts
10 oz (1 pkg) Chopped Spinach (frozen)
1/3 medium Yellow Onion, diced
1/2 tsp Garlic Powder
1/4 tsp Kosher Salt
1/2 tsp Ground Black Pepper
8 oz Mushrooms (button), sliced
1 cup (dry) Brown Rice
1 tsp Minced Garlic
3/4 cup Shredded Part-skim Mozzarella Cheese

NUTRITION FACTS	
Serving Size: 1/6 casserole	
Amount per Serving	
Calories 294	Calories from Fat 55.2
	% Daily Value *
Total Fat 6.13g	9%
Saturated Fat 2.28g	11%
Cholesterol 72.5mg	24%
Sodium 498.74mg	20%
Total Carbohydrate 27.72g	9%
Dietary Fiber 2.49g	9%
Sugars 1.13g	
Protein 31.64g	63%

Directions:
Cook rice and spinach as directed on packaging. Drain spinach well after cooking. Sauté diced onions and minced garlic until softened. Cut up raw chicken into small chunks, and cook with garlic powder and stir in skillet until white & done. Spray baking dish with nonstick spray. Preheat oven to 350F.
Evenly spread cooked rice across bottom of baking dish. Mix onions and minced garlic with spinach, then spread mixture over rice. Arrange mushrooms evenly over spinach mixture. Place chicken chunks over mushrooms. Sprinkle cheese evenly over top of casserole.
Bake in preheated oven for 20-30 minutes until cheese is completely melted & beginning to brown.

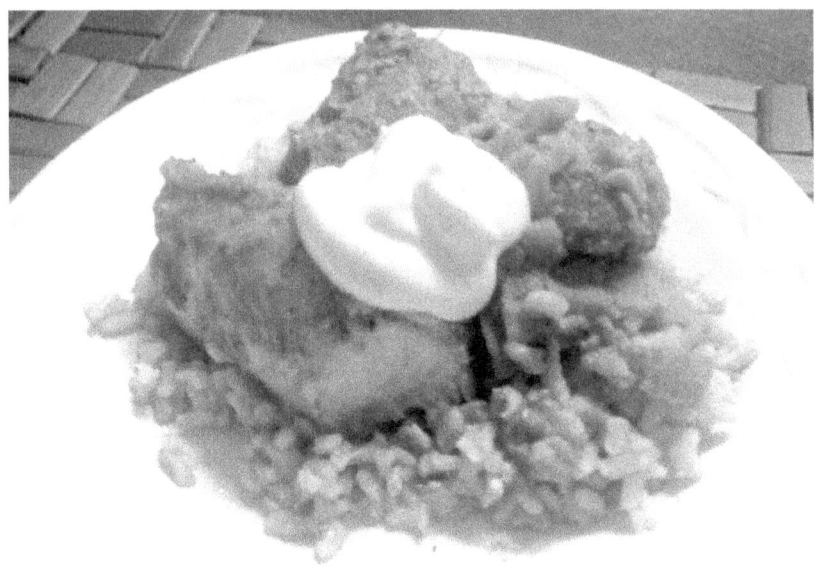

Saucy Mexican Chicken & Rice

NUTRITION FACTS

Serving Size: 1 breast

Amount per Serving

Calories 350   Calories from Fat 81.5

% Daily Value *

Total Fat 9.05g	13%
Saturated Fat 7.83g	39%
Cholesterol 68.33mg	22%
Sodium 464.93mg	19%
Total Carbohydrate 36.6g	12%
Dietary Fiber 2.27g	9%
Sugars 1.33g	
Protein 29.3g	58%

Saucy Mexican Chicken & Rice

Time: 50 minutes
Servings: 6 (1 breast & ½ cup cooked rice each)

Ingredients:
28 oz boneless skinless chicken breasts (6 med)
½ cup medium chunky salsa
¼ cup Dijon-style mustard
2 tbsp lime juice
2 tsp Ground Cumin
8 tbsp Reduced Fat Sour Cream
1 1/2 cups (dry) Brown Rice

Directions:
Start preparing rice as directed on packaging. Sprinkle in 1 tsp of cumin in water with rice. Allow to cook/ simmer.
Combine salsa, mustard, lime juice, & 1 tsp cumin in large bowl. Place chicken in bowl, and toss to coat well. Cover and marinate for 30 minutes (while rice is cooking).
Use large non-stick skillet & spray with nonstick spray - bring to med-high heat. Remove chicken from marinade BUT save marinade to the side. Place chicken in heated skillet, cooking about 10 minutes, or until both sides are browned. Add in reserved marinade to skillet with chicken. Cook with marinade about 5-10 minutes until chicken is thoroughly cooked & glazed in marinade. Remove chicken from skillet, and boil marinade for about 1 minute over high heat.
Serve chicken over rice. Evenly pour remaining marinade over chicken, and top with sour cream.

Tart Cherry Chicken & Rice

Time: 45 minutes
Servings: 6 (1 chicken breast, 1/6th sauce mix,
& 2/3 cup cooked rice each)

NUTRITION FACTS	
Serving Size: 1 breast	
Amount per Serving	
Calories 353	Calories from Fat 49.8
	% Daily Value *
Total Fat 5.53g	8%
Saturated Fat 1.86g	9%
Cholesterol 86.25mg	28%
Sodium 323.61mg	13%
Total Carbohydrate 44.11g	14%
Dietary Fiber 2.83g	11%
Sugars 14.97g	
Protein 33.81g	67%

Ingredients:
30 oz boneless skinless chicken breasts (6 med)
2 tbsp Whipped Butter
2 cups Pitted Canned Tart Cherries in Light Syrup
(undrained)
1 tbsp Pure Cornstarch
2 tbsp Worcestershire Sauce
1 1/2 tsp Light Brown Sugar
2 tsp Minced Garlic
1/3 medium Yellow Onion, finely diced
2 cups (dry) Wild Rice (to make 4 cups cooked)

Tart Cherry Chicken & Rice (cont'd)

Directions:
(Optional: Salt & pepper to taste)
Preheat oven to 350F. Spray baking dish with nonstick spray. Option: lightly sprinkle chicken with salt, and generously with pepper. Heat butter over med-high heat in large skillet. Add chicken and cook 5-7 mins per side, or until browned. Remove chicken from skillet, and place in baking dish.
Drain cherries from can, saving about 1/4 cup juice. Add juice to skillet, and stir in cornstarch well.
In food processor or blender, combine 1 cup cherries (reserve the rest), Worcestershire sauce, sugar, and garlic. Blend until smooth, and add to skillet (with cornstarch mix). Stir in remaining cherries and onion. Cook over med-high heat 3-4 minutes until sauce begins to boil and thicken, stirring constantly. Evenly pour sauce over chicken in baking dish. Meanwhile, cook rice as directed on packaging.
Bake chicken 20-30 minutes until thoroughly cooked. Serve chicken over rice, and drizzle sauce over chicken and rice.

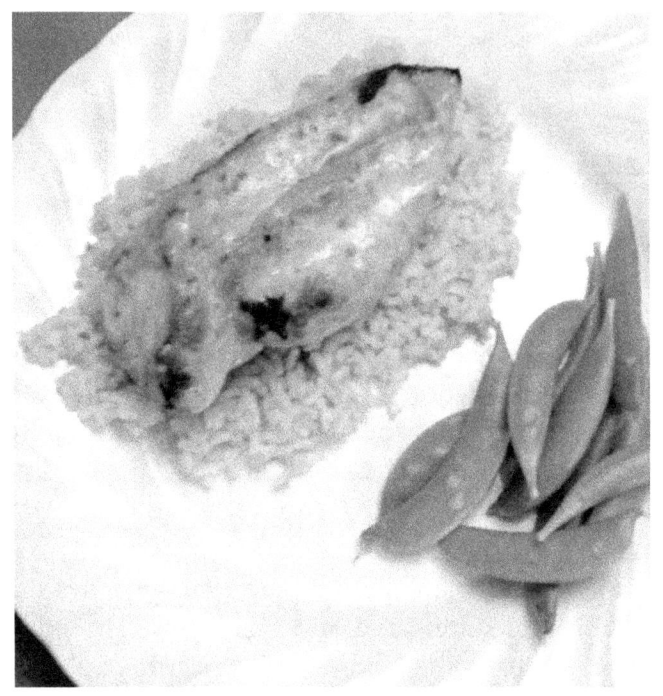

Chinese BBQ Chicken

NUTRITION FACTS

Serving Size: 1 breast

Amount per Serving

Calories 365	Calories from Fat 52.9

	% Daily Value *
Total Fat 5.88g	9%
Saturated Fat 1.25g	6%
Cholesterol 62.5mg	20%
Sodium 658.75mg	27%
Total Carbohydrate 44.83g	14%
Dietary Fiber 2g	8%
Sugars 8g	
Protein 31.25g	62%

Chinese BBQ Chicken

Time: 45 minutes
Servings: 6 (1 breast & ½ cup cooked rice each)

Ingredients:
30 oz boneless skinless chicken breast (6 med)
12 oz Pineapple Juice, Unsweetened
3 tbsp Reduced Sodium Soy Sauce
1 tbsp Minced Garlic
1 tsp Chinese Five Spice Powder
1 1/2 tsp 100% Pure Cornstarch
1 1/2 cups (dry) Brown Rice

Directions:
Begin cooking rice as directed on packaging.
In small bowl, combine juice, spices, soy sauce, and garlic. Place chicken in large plastic bag with zipper top. Add juice & marinate chicken at least 20 minutes, or overnight.
Drain marinade into small sauce pan, and stir in cornstarch. Cook over med-high heat until sauce begins to boil and thicken. Meanwhile, place marinated chicken on greased broiler pan (or grill). Broil 4-5" from heat (or grill) for 10-15 minutes on each side or until chicken is tender & cooked thoroughly. While chicken is broiling or grilling, baste often with marinade.
Serve chicken over rice. (Alternate preparation: Instead of rice, shred chicken when done, and serve on whole wheat buns.)

Turkey Taco Loaded Potato Skins

Time: 30-45 minutes
Servings: 6

Ingredients:
1 lb ground turkey
3 Idaho Potatoes
1/3 medium Yellow
Onion, chopped
2 tsp Minced Garlic
8 oz (1 can) Stewed
Tomatoes
2 tsp Chili Powder
1/2 tsp Ground Cumin
1/4 tbsp Dried
Oregano
1/4 tsp Crushed Red Pepper
1/4 tsp Kosher Salt
1/3 cup Reduced Fat Shredded Cheddar

NUTRITION FACTS	
Serving Size: 1 loaded skin	
Amount per Serving	
Calories 205	Calories from Fat 59.7
	% Daily Value *
Total Fat 6.63g	10%
Saturated Fat 2.37g	11%
Cholesterol 56.66mg	18%
Sodium 357.35mg	14%
Total Carbohydrate 16.78g	5%
Dietary Fiber 1.93g	7%
Sugars 2.94g	
Protein 17.58g	35%

Directions:
Bake potatoes, then cool and set aside (this can be done in advance). Keep oven preheated to 375F.
Cut potatoes in half length-wise, and scoop centers to within about 1/4" of bottom and sides (reserve potato insides for use at a later time, if desired).
In large skillet over med-high heat, combine ground turkey, onion, and garlic. Cook until turkey is no longer pink (drain if needed). Add tomatoes with juice, and all spices and herbs. Simmer, stirring occasionally, for about 15 minutes most of the liquid is absorbed.
Evenly distribute turkey mix into potato halves, and sprinkle evenly with cheese. Place loaded skins in baking dish, and bake for about 15 minutes until cheese is melted.

13. RECIPES: SLOW COOKERS

If recipe does not call for a serving of green veggies and/ or a carb, add it to the side for a complete meal! Refer to Snacks & Sides List for ideas.

Check "Servings:" in Recipes for correct servings sizes versus Nutrition Label

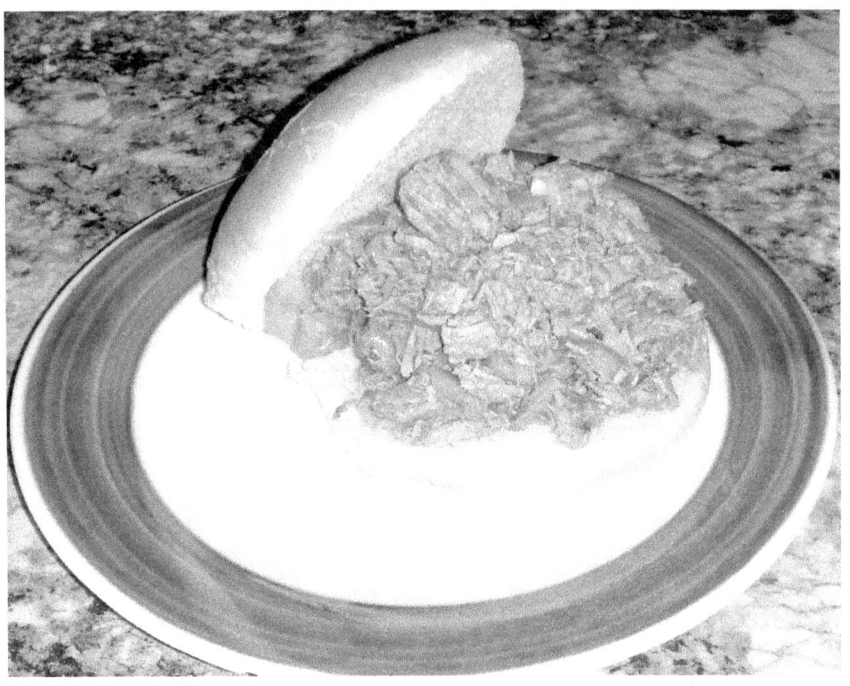

Italian Beef Sandwiches

NUTRITION FACTS

Serving Size: 1 sandwhiches

Amount per Serving

Calories 271 — Calories from Fat 65.3

	% Daily Value *
Total Fat 7.26g	11%
Saturated Fat 1.92g	9%
Cholesterol 72mg	24%
Sodium 555.4mg	23%
Total Carbohydrate 20.7g	6%
Dietary Fiber 1g	4%
Sugars 2g	
Protein 28g	56%

Italian Beef Sandwiches

Time: 4-8 hours
Servings: 10

Ingredients:
1 large jar sliced Golden Pepperoncinis (undrained)
2.5 lb Rump Roast
10 Whole Wheat Hamburger Bun

Directions:
Put roast in slow cooker. Cover with whole jar of peppers and liquid (16 oz. from jar, then 1.5 jar-fulls of water.
Cook on high for about 3-5 hrs, or low for about 7-9 hrs. (Low and slow is best for tender meat)
Pull meat from liquid (do NOT drain!), shred beef, then add meat back to liquid and peppers and stir well. Strain meat and peppers from liquid. Serve on a whole wheat bun with green veggie on the side.

Turkey Chili

Time: 4 or 8 hours
Servings: 6

```
NUTRITION FACTS
Serving Size: 2 1/3 cup

Amount per Serving
Calories 404              Calories from Fat 108.7

                                    % Daily Value *

Total Fat 12.08g                              18%
    Saturated Fat 3.33g                       16%
Cholesterol 106.67mg                          35%
Sodium 975.83mg                               40%
Total Carbohydrate 26.5g                       8%
    Dietary Fiber 8.13g                       32%
    Sugars 7.71g
Protein 42.21g                                84%
```

Ingredients:
2 lb Ground Turkey
2 2/3 tbsp Chili Seasoning
29 oz Diced Tomatoes
15 oz Dark Red Kidney Beans
15 oz Light Red Kidney Beans
2 cups Water

Directions:
Add/ stir meat and all ingredients (don't drain juice from cans) in slow cooker very well. Cook on high 4 hours or low 8 hours.

New YOU Clam Chowder

Time: 8 hrs
Servings: 6

Ingredients:
1 medium raw Yellow
Onion, diced
5 red potatoes, cut into
1" cubes
6 1/2 oz (1 small can)
Minced Clams (drained)
5 slices Low Sodium
Turkey Bacon, chopped
& browned
1 stalk of celery, minced
1 tbsp Minced Garlic
2 tsp dried Thyme
4 cups water
4 tsp Chicken Flavor
Instant Bouillon
Granules
1 tsp Kosher Salt
1 tsp Ground Black Pepper
2 cups Unsweetened Vanilla Almond Milk
1 cup Mild Shredded Reduced Fat Cheddar Cheese

NUTRITION FACTS	
Serving Size: 1/6 crock pot	
Amount per Serving	
Calories 184	Calories from Fat 46.2
	% Daily Value '
Total Fat 5.13g	7%
Saturated Fat 2.42g	12%
Cholesterol 26.46mg	8%
Sodium 1234.58mg	51%
Total Carbohydrate 25.07g	8%
Dietary Fiber 3.4g	13%
Sugars 3.79g	
Protein 14.66g	29%
Est. Percent of Calories from:	
Fat	25%
Carbs	54%
Protein	31%

Directions:
Add clams, vegetables, and spices to slow cooker. Mix 4 cups of
warm water and granules to create broth and pour in slow
cooker.
Cover, and cook on low for about 8 hours, or until the onion
and potatoes are tender. Mix gently to thicken the soup, then
add in almond milk and shredded cheese and stir well.

Apples & Cider Pork Pot Roast

Time: 4 hrs on low OR 8 hrs on high
Serving: 5

Ingredients:
1 large Yellow Onion
2 lb Extra Lean
Boneless Pork
Shoulder Picnic
Roast
4 medium Apples,
Red Delicious
12 oz baby carrots
1 tbsp Minced Garlic
1/2 tsp Coarse
Kosher Salt
1/2 tsp Pure Ground
Black Pepper
1 tsp Allspice,
Ground
1 tsp Thyme, Dried
2 tbsp Apple Cider Vinegar
16 oz Light Apple Juice

NUTRITION FACTS	
Serving Size: 1/5 roast and veggies	
Amount per Serving	
Calories 333	Calories from Fat 65.4
	% Daily Value *
Total Fat 7.27g	11%
Saturated Fat 2.41g	12%
Cholesterol 96mg	32%
Sodium 598.43mg	24%
Total Carbohydrate 34.01g	11%
Dietary Fiber 5.77g	23%
Sugars 25.08g	
Protein 34.44g	68%

Directions:
Slice and arrange onions in the bottom of the slow cooker.
Place roast in the slow cooker.
Arrange carrots around the roast; sprinkle the roast with the
garlic, salt, pepper, allspice, and thyme. Core and cut apples into
quarters and place on top of roast. Combine the juice and
vinegar and pour over the roast.
Cover and cook on LOW and cook for 6 to 8 hours longer, or
leave on HIGH for 3 to 4 hours longer.

Jerk Chicken & Brown Rice

Time: 8 hrs
Servings: 5

Ingredients:
5 med Boneless
Skinless Chicken
Breasts (approx 25
oz)
1 1/4 cups Brown
Rice
3 cups water
1 tbsp Caribbean
Jerk Seasoning
1 cup Sliced Buttons
Mushrooms
2 tsp Chicken
Flavor Instant
Bouillion Granules

NUTRITION FACTS

Serving Size : 1 breast and rice

Amount per Serving

Calories 318   Calories from Fat 41.7

	% Daily Value *
Total Fat 4.63g	7%
Saturated Fat 0.63g	3%
Cholesterol 81.25mg	27%
Sodium 850.4mg	35%
Total Carbohydrate 36.6g	12%
Dietary Fiber 2.4g	9%
Sugars 0.4g	
Protein 33.55g	67%

Directions:
Spray inside of slow cooker with nonstick spray. Whisk
granules, seasoning and water well, then whisk in rice and pour
in slow cooker. Place 5 med chicken breasts in slow cooker on
top of rice mixture.
Set to low for 6-7 hours. Fluff rice with fork before serving.

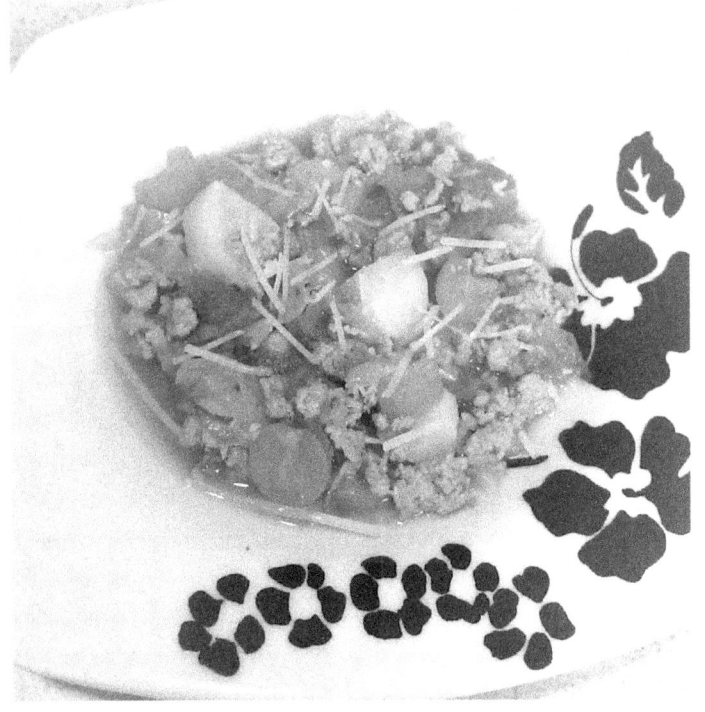

<u>Turkey Minestrone Soup</u>

NUTRITION FACTS

Serving Size: 1/6 pot of soup

Amount per Serving

Calories 182	Calories from Fat 70.0
	% Daily Value *
Total Fat 7.78g	**11%**
Saturated Fat 1.84g	**9%**
Cholesterol 69.17mg	**23%**
Sodium 781.58mg	**32%**
Total Carbohydrate 15.31g	**5%**
Dietary Fiber 2.76g	**11%**
Sugars 3.08g	
Protein 19.11g	**38%**

Turkey Minestrone Soup

Time: 3-12 hours
Servings: 6

Ingredients:
1 lb Ground Turkey
2 Whole Carrots
2 celery stalks
1 medium Yellow Onion
1 cup shredded cabbage
2 Idaho potatoes
1 can (20 oz) whole tomatoes
1 tsp Coarse Kosher Salt
1/2 tsp Thyme, Dried
1/2 tsp Basil, Dried
1/2 tsp Ground Black Pepper
2 tsp Beef Flavor Bouillon
3 tbsp Parmesan Cheese-grated

Directions:
Chop onion & celery. Slice carrots. Peel and cube potatoes. Add all ingredients EXCEPT cheese to slow cooker. Cover all ingredients with water.
Cover and set to cook on low for 8-12 hours, or high for 3-5 hours. Stir well. Serve with sprinkled parmesan cheese on top.

Harvest Turkey & Sweet Potatoes

Time: 8 hrs on low
Servings: 6

Ingredients:
2 lb Boneless Turkey
Breast
4 medium Sweet
Potato
1 medium , raw Yellow
Onion
1 tbsp Allspice,
Ground
1 tbsp Spices,
Cinnamon, Ground
1 tbsp Cloves, Ground
2 tbsp Salted Whipped
Butter
2 cups water

NUTRITION FACTS	
Serving Size: 1/6 breast and potatoes	
Amount per Serving	
Calories 261	Calories from Fat 26.7
	% Daily Value *
Total Fat 2.97g	4%
Saturated Fat 1.27g	6%
Cholesterol 98.33mg	32%
Sodium 123.93mg	5%
Total Carbohydrate 19.88g	6%
Dietary Fiber 4.25g	17%
Sugars 14.58g	
Protein 39.01g	78%
Est. Percent of Calories from:	
Fat	10%
Carbs	30%
Protein	59%

Directions:
Spray inside of slow cooker. Rough chop onion and place in
bottom of slow cooker. Place raw breast on top of onion. Peel
& cut up sweet potatoes into large cubes (approx 1.5") and
place evenly on top of breast.
Melt butter and whisk with water and spices. Pour over
everything in slow cooker. Set to low and cook for 8 hours.

Sausage & Rice Casserole

Time: 3-9 hours
Servings: 6

Ingredients:
14 oz. smoked
turkey sausage, cut
into ½" chunks
1 1/2 cups (dry)
Brown Rice
3 tsp Chicken flavor
Bouillon Granules
1/3 cup Slivered
Almonds
4 cups water
2 tsp Dried Thyme
2 tsp Garlic Powder
1 tbsp Minced
Onions

NUTRITION FACTS

Serving Size: 1/6 crockpot

Amount per Serving

Calories 326	Calories from Fat 104.8
	% Daily Value *
Total Fat 11.64g	17%
Saturated Fat 2.56g	12%
Cholesterol 35mg	11%
Sodium 1090.22mg	45%
Total Carbohydrate 41.7g	13%
Dietary Fiber 2.8g	11%
Sugars 1.39g	
Protein 14.7g	29%

Directions
Heat large skillet to med-high heat and brown sausage chunks.
Drain well.
Lightly grease slow cooker. Add all ingredients to slow cooker
and stir well. Cover and cook on low 7-9 hours, OR on high 3-4
hours (until rice is tender). Fluff with a fork and stir before
serving.

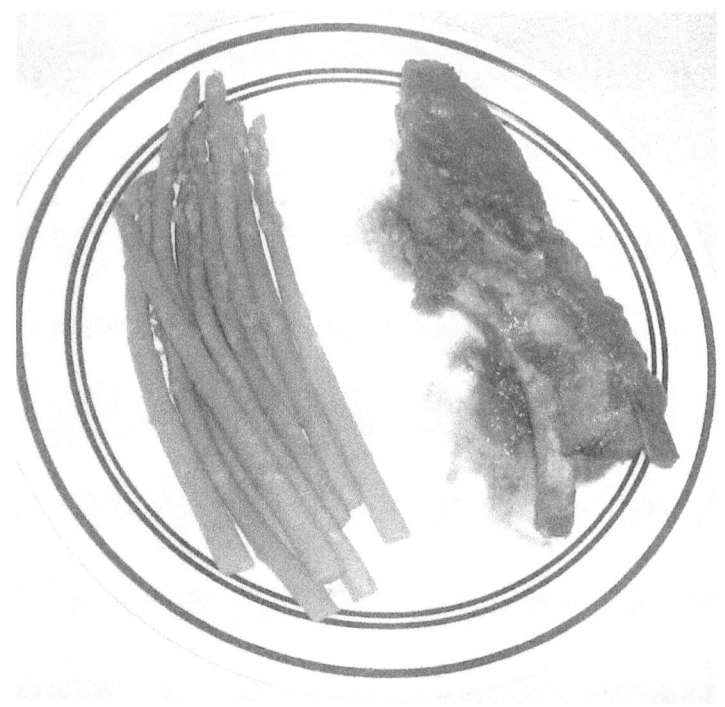

<u>Orange-Spiced Spare Ribs</u>

NUTRITION FACTS

Serving Size: 1/6 crock pot

Amount per Serving

Calories 425   Calories from Fat 183.3

	% Daily Value *
Total Fat 20.37g	31%
Saturated Fat 6.34g	31%
Cholesterol 100mg	33%
Sodium 1286.91mg	53%
Total Carbohydrate 20.05g	6%
Dietary Fiber 2.06g	8%
Sugars 15g	
Protein 47.45g	94%

Orange-Spiced Spare Ribs

Time: 5-7 hours
Servings: 6

Ingredients:
3 lb Country Style Pork Spare Ribs
1 tbsp Vegetable Oil
1 medium Yellow Onion, thinly sliced
2 tsp Chili Powder
1/2 tsp Cinnamon, Ground
1/4 tsp Cloves, Ground
1 can Crushed Tomatoes, canned, undrained
2 tsp Garlic Minced
1/2 cup Light Orange Juice
1/4 cup Light Brown Sugar
1/2 orange (medium)
1/4 tsp Coarse Kosher Salt
1 tbsp Cider vinegar

Directions:
Peel orange, separate sections, and thinly shred peel. Trim excess fat from ribs & cut into individual riblets. Heat oil in large skillet to medium heat. Brown riblets for about 10 minutes or until brown on all sides. Set to the side. Add onion slices, chili powder, cinnamon, and cloves into slow cooker.
Add remaining ingredients including orange peel (EXCEPT for riblets, orange sections, & vinegar) to slow cooker over onion mixture. Add ribs to mixture, and stir to coat with sauce. Add orange sections on top.
Cover and cook on low 5-6 hours until riblets are tender. Remove ribs from slow cooker and set aside. Pour juice from slow cooker into large bowl and let stand for 5 minutes. Skim any fat from top. Stir in vinegar to juice, and serve over riblets and any accompanying sides if desired.

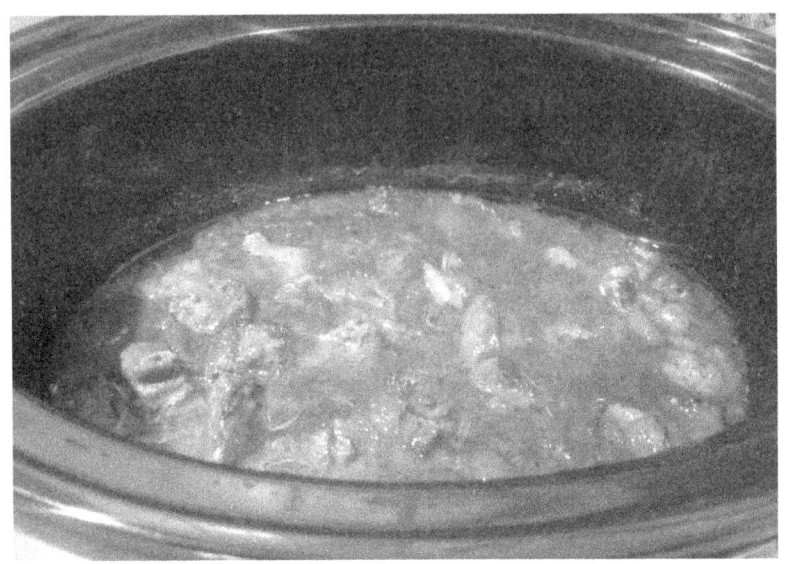

Pork Stew & Rice

NUTRITION FACTS

Serving Size: 1/7 crockpot

Amount per Serving

Calories 351	Calories from Fat 71.7

	% Daily Value *
Total Fat 7.97g	12%
Saturated Fat 1.91g	9%
Cholesterol 68.57mg	22%
Sodium 930.78mg	38%
Total Carbohydrate 40.84g	13%
Dietary Fiber 3.7g	14%
Sugars 4.15g	
Protein 28.29g	56%

Pork Stew & Rice

Time: 4-9 hours
Servings: 7

Ingredients:
2 lb Lean Boneless Pork Shoulder Picnic Roast
2 tsp Extra Virgin Olive Oil
2 medium White Onion
1 tbsp Minced Garlic
1 tsp Coarse Kosher Salt
1 tsp Ground Cumin
1 tsp dried oregano
1 tsp dried basil
1 can Stewed Tomatoes
1 small can Chopped Green Chilies
4 tsp Red. Sodium Chicken Flavor Bouillon Granules
1/2 tsp Ground Coriander
2 tsp Lime Juice
1 1/2 cups (dry) Brown Rice

Directions:
Cut pork into ½ inch chunks. Thinly slice onions. Heat oil to med-high heat and brown pork chunks for 8-10 minutes or until browned on all sides. Remove pork from skillet and set aside. Add onions, salt, cumin, garlic, oregano, basil, coriander, and browned pork (EXCEPT RICE) to slow cooker and add 1.5 cups of water. Cover and cook on low for 7-9 hours OR on high for 4-5 hours.
Meanwhile, cook rice as directed on packaging. Serve pork stew over rice.

Turkey Meatballs & Gravy

Time: 4 – 10 hours
Servings: 6
(1 serving = 5 meatballs, 1/6 gravy, 1 cup cooked pasta)

Ingredients:
30 frozen turkey
meatballs (6 servings)
1 tsp Extra Virgin
Olive Oil
1 can (10 ¾ oz) 98%
Fat Free Cream of
Mushroom Soup
1 cup water
1 packet (24g) Turkey
Gravy Mix
1 tbsp Italian
Seasoning
1 tsp Lemon Juice
12 oz (dry) Veggie
Rotini (about 1 box)
1 tbsp Whipped Butter

NUTRITION FACTS

Serving Size: 5 meatballs

Amount per Serving
Calories 459   Calories from Fat 119.9

	% Daily Value *
Total Fat 13.32g	20%
Saturated Fat 0.92g	4%
Cholesterol 4.74mg	1%
Sodium 525.41mg	21%
Total Carbohydrate 50.28g	16%
Dietary Fiber 3.12g	12%
Sugars 3.11g	
Protein 32.6g	65%

Directions:
Heat oil in large skillet to med-high heat. Add frozen meatballs
to skillet and brown (8-10 minutes). Add meatballs to slow
cooker.
In large bowl, mix soup, water, gravy mix, seasoning, and lemon
juice. Pour over meatballs. Cover and cook on low 6-8 hours
OR on high 3-4 hours.
Meanwhile, cook noodles as directed on package. Drain. Toss
with 1 tbsp butter. Serve meatballs and gravy over buttered
veggie noodles.

"Holy Garlic!" Chicken

Time: 7-9 hours
Servings: 6

Ingredients:
3 lb whole chicken
1 tbsp Extra Virgin
Olive Oil
1/3 cup white wine
vinegar
1/3 cup Light White
Grape Juice
1 tbsp Italian Seasoning
1/2 tsp red pepper
flakes
40 garlic cloves (about 2 heads), peeled
3 large celery stalks, sliced
1 whole Lemon

NUTRITION FACTS	
Serving Size 5 1/3 oz	
Amount per Serving	
Calories 325	Calories from Fat 132 4
	% Daily Value *
Total Fat 14 71g	22%
Saturated Fat 3 73g	18%
Cholesterol 158 34mg	52%
Sodium 1071 08mg	44%
Total Carbohydrate 12 67g	4%
Dietary Fiber 2g	8%
Sugars 3 83g	
Protein 37 54g	75%

Directions:
Remove skin from chicken and cut into serving pieces. Sprinkle with salt & pepper (if desired). Heat oil in large skillet to med-high heat. Add chicken and rotate and cook about 10 minutes or until browned on all sides. Remove chicken and drain oil. Mix vinegar, grape juice, Italian seasoning, and red pepper flakes in large bowl. Add garlic cloves and celery slices and mix well. With slotted spoon, remove garlic and celery from bowl and add to slow cooker. Add chicken to herb/ juice mixture and coat well. Place chicken on top of garlic and celery in slow cooker. Juice and peel lemon; evenly pour juice in slow cooker, then add peel. Evenly pour remaining herb/ juice mix to slow cooker.
Cover & cook on low 7-9 hours (until chicken is no longer pink in center). Remove skin before serving to reduce fat.

Mediterranean Chicken & Veggie Stew

Time: 4 – 10 hours
Servings: 6 (1 serving = 1/6 pot of stew, 1 cup cooked couscous)

Ingredients:
20 oz Chicken Breast (boneless,skinless), cut into half-inch cubes
24 oz Butternut Squash, cut into one-inch cubes
1 1/4 lb Eggplant [medium], cut into one-inch cubes
1 can (15 ½ oz) Chickpeas (garbanzo Beans), drained
1 can (8 oz) Tomato Sauce
1 medium Yellow Onions, chopped
1 medium Tomato, chopped
1 Large Carrot, sliced
1/2 tsp Sodium Free Chicken Bouillon
1/2 cup water
1/4 cup Raisins
1 tsp Minced Garlic
1 tsp ground cumin
3/4 tsp Ground Turmeric
1/2 tsp Red Pepper Flakes
1/2 tsp Ground Cinnamon
1/2 tsp Paprika
2 cups (dry) Wheat Couscous

NUTRITION FACTS	
Serving Size: 1/6 pot stew	
Amount per Serving	
Calories 475	Calories from Fat 46.4
	% Daily Value *
Total Fat 5.15g	7%
Saturated Fat 0.47g	2%
Cholesterol 54.17mg	18%
Sodium 346.6mg	14%
Total Carbohydrate 79.69g	26%
Dietary Fiber 12.11g	48%
Sugars 16.49g	
Protein 34.35g	68%

Mediterranean Chicken & Veggie Stew (cont'd)

Directions:

Add all ingredients EXCEPT couscous to slow cooker and mix well. Cover and cook on low 8-10 hours or until vegetables are tender.

Prepare couscous as directed on package. (Makes about 6 cups cooked couscous)

Serve stew over couscous.

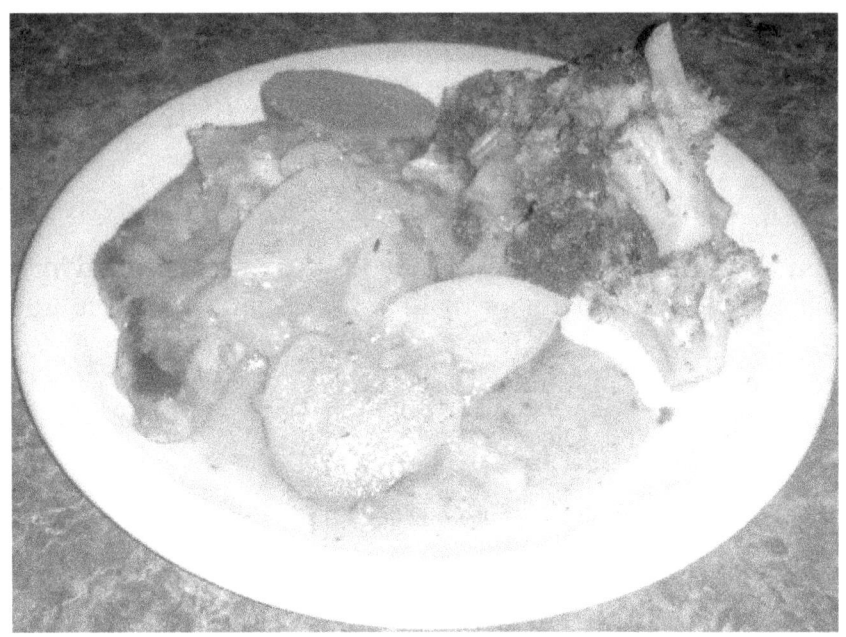

<u>Saucy Mustard Pork Chops & Potatoes</u>

NUTRITION FACTS	
Serving Size: 1 chop and potatoes	
Amount per Serving	
Calories 333	Calories from Fat 95.0
	% Daily Value *
Total Fat 10.55g	**16%**
Saturated Fat 3.44g	**17%**
Cholesterol 53.54mg	**17%**
Sodium 875.48mg	**36%**
Total Carbohydrate 27.24g	**9%**
Dietary Fiber 4.18g	**16%**
Sugars 4.75g	
Protein 27.47g	**54%**

Saucy Mustard Pork Chops & Potatoes

Time: 4 – 10 hours
Servings: 6

Ingredients:
1.7 lb Boneless Pork Top Loin Chops (6 4-5oz chops)
1 tbsp Extra Virgin Olive Oil
1 can 98% Fat Free Cream of Mushroom Soup
1 tsp Sodium Free Chicken Bouillon Granules
1.5 cup water
1/3 cup Dijon Mustard
3/4 tsp Dried Thyme
1/2 tsp Garlic Powder
1/2 tsp Ground Black Pepper
5 Idaho Potatoes, sliced into ½" slices
1 medium Yellow Onion, thinly sliced

Directions:
Heat oil in skillet to med-high heat, and brown pork chops on both sides until light brown. Remove chops & drain well.
In slow cooker, whisk soup, chicken granules, water, mustard, thyme, garlic powder, & pepper. Add slices of potatoes and onion, and stir to coat with mixture. Add pork chops on top of mixture in slow cooker. Cover and cook on low 8-10 hours OR high 4-5 hours.

14. RECIPES: DESSERTS

Check "Servings:" in Recipes for correct servings sizes versus Nutrition Label

Ashley's Banana Bread

Time: 75 mins
Servings: 8 (slices)

Ingredients:
2 large Egg Whites
1 1/3 cups Whole
Wheat Flour
4 tbsp Whipped Butter
2 tsp Ground Allspice
2 tsp Cinnamon
1 tsp Ground Cloves
3/4 tsp Sea Salt
3/4 tsp Baking Soda
1/4 tsp Baking
Powder
1/4 cup Light Brown
Sugar
1/2 cup Granulated No Calorie Sweetener
2 tbsp Ground Flaxseed
2 medium ripe Bananas
1 tbsp Chopped Walnuts
2 tsp Pure Vanilla Extract
1/4 cup Unsweetened Almond Milk

NUTRITION FACTS	
Serving Size: 1/8 loaf	
Amount per Serving	
Calories 160	Calories from Fat 43.7
	% Daily Value *
Total Fat 4.86g	7%
Saturated Fat 1.91g	9%
Cholesterol 7.5mg	2%
Sodium 287.96mg	11%
Total Carbohydrate 28.89g	9%
Dietary Fiber 3.8g	15%
Sugars 11.6g	
Protein 4.43g	8%

Directions:
Preheat oven to 350. Grease/ spray bread pan. Soften butter (in microwave for 10-15 seconds). Beat egg whites and mash bananas separately.

In large bowl, stir flour, baking soda, baking powder, allspice, cinnamon, flaxseed, and salt.

In separate bowl, cream butter/ margarine, splenda, milk, and sugar. Then add in beaten eggs and mashed bananas. Stir in vanilla extract.

Fold banana mix into flour mix - stir just to moisten. Pour into bread pan. Then sprinkle evenly with walnuts. Bake about 55 minutes.

Easy Peach Cobbler

Time: 55 mins
Servings: 8

Ingredients:
1/3 cup Salted
Whipped Butter
1 cup Specialty Flour
Whole Wheat
1 cup Granulated
Baking Splenda
1/3 cup Light Brown
Sugar®
1 3/4 tsp Baking
Powder
3/4 cup Fat Free
Skim Milk
29 oz (2 reg cans –
drained) No Sugar
Added Sliced Peaches
2 tsp Pure Vanilla
Extract

NUTRITION FACTS	
Serving Size: 1/8 cobbler	
Amount per Serving	
Calories 168	Calories from Fat 38.3
	% Daily Value *
Total Fat 4.25g	6%
Saturated Fat 2.33g	11%
Cholesterol 10.46mg	3%
Sodium 159.55mg	6%
Total Carbohydrate 32.93g	10%
Dietary Fiber 3.31g	13%
Sugars 16.62g	
Protein 3.75g	7%
Est. Percent of Calories from:	
Fat	21%
Carbs	78%
Protein	8%

Directions:
Preheat oven to 350. Spray sides of 8x8 glass baking dish with nonstick spray, then add butter to bottom of pan, place in oven, and melt for about 5 minutes.

Meanwhile in mixing bowl, mix flour, sugar, sweetener, baking powder, and vanilla. When smooth, fold in peaches (drained from can).

Pour mix over hot melted butter in dish. Bake in oven for 45 mins until brown on top and crispy at edges. Let cool and set for 5-10 minutes before cutting and serving.

Triple Chocolate Pot O'Heaven (Slow Cooker)

Time: 3-4 hours
Servings: 12 (1/12th of cake/ slow cooker)

Ingredients:
1 package Sugar Free Devil's Food Cake Mix
1/3 cup Light Sour Cream
1 pkg Sugar Free Chocolate Pudding Mix
3/4 cup Granulated
No Calorie Sweetener
2/3 cup Dark
Chocolate Chip
Morsels
1 cup Unsweetened
Apple Sauce
3 large Egg Whites
1 egg
1 cup water

Directions:
Spray slow cooker
with non-stick
spray. In large bowl,
mix all ingredients
well. Pour batter into crock-pot. Cover and cook on low 6-8
hours OR on high 3-4 hours.

NUTRITION FACTS	
Serving Size: 0 cake	
Amount per Serving	
Calories 215	Calories from Fat 77.6
	% Daily Value *
Total Fat 8.62g	13%
Saturated Fat 0.57g	2%
Cholesterol 17.64mg	5%
Sodium 337.83mg	14%
Total Carbohydrate 41.01g	13%
Dietary Fiber 2.22g	8%
Sugars 9.12g	
Protein 3.84g	7%

Spicy Pumpkin Bread

Time: 75 mins
Servings: 16 (2 loaves – 8 slices each)

Ingredients:
4 cups Specialty Flour Whole Wheat
½ cup Light Brown Sugar & No-Calorie Sweetener Blend
2 tsp Baking Soda
2 tsp Baking Powder
15 oz Pumpkin
1 tbsp Allspice, Ground
1 tbsp Cinnamon, Ground
2 large Egg White
14 oz Light Pulp Free Orange Juice
1/2 cup Raw Chopped Walnuts

NUTRITION FACTS	
Serving Size. 1/8 loaves	
Amount per Serving	
Calories 161	Calories from Fat 26.7
	% Daily Value *
Total Fat 2.97g	4%
Saturated Fat 0.2g	1%
Cholesterol 0mg	0%
Sodium 219.64mg	9%
Total Carbohydrate 31.71g	10%
Dietary Fiber 4.69g	18%
Sugars 8.19g	
Protein 5.44g	10%

Directions:
Preheat oven to 350°F.

In a large bowl, combine the flour, sugar, baking soda, baking powder, allspice, and cinnamon, then stir to mix well. Add the orange juice, pumpkin, and egg white, and stir just until the dry ingredients are moistened. Fold in the walnuts.

Spray two 9x5 loaf pans with non-stick spray. Spread the batter in the pans equally, and bake at 350°F for 45 minutes, or until a wooden toothpick inserted in the center comes out clean.

Remove the bread from the oven, and let sit for 10 minutes. Invert the loaf onto a wire rack, turn right side up, and cool to room temperature before slicing.

Spicy Pear Crisp

Time: 35 mins
Servings: 12

Ingredients:
4 14.5 oz cans No
Sugar Added Sliced
Pears
1 cup Specialty Flour
Whole Wheat
2 cups 100% Whole
Grain Quick Oats
1/2 cup Light Brown
Sugar
1 cup Granulated
Splenda
2 tbsp Ground
Cinnamon
4 tsp Ground Allspice
1 tsp Coarse Kosher
Salt
2/3 cup Salted
Whipped Butter

NUTRITION FACTS
Serving Size: 0 dish

Amount per Serving
Calories 207   Calories from Fat 58.9

	% Daily Value *
Total Fat 6.54g	10%
Saturated Fat 3.3g	16%
Cholesterol 13.34mg	4%
Sodium 214.98mg	8%
Total Carbohydrate 35.36g	11%
Dietary Fiber 4.09g	16%
Sugars 17.38g	
Protein 3.08g	6%

Est. Percent of Calories from:	
Fat	26%
Carbs	68%
Protein	5%

Directions:
Preheat oven to 400. Cut pear slices in half. Spray 9x13" glass baking dish with nonstick spray. Put drained and cut pear slices in bottom of dish.
Melt butter. Mix oats, spices, flour, sugar, splenda, and salt in bowl. Add melted butter and blend well with fork to a crumble. Sprinkle over fruit and bake 25-30 mins. Let cool and set 5-10 mins before cutting and serving.

Fruity & Nutty Baked Apples (Slow Cooker)

Time: 3-4 hours
Servings: 4

Ingredients:
4 apple, large-sized, with skin
1 tbsp Lemon Juice
8 pieces Dried Apricots, chopped
3 tbsp - Chopped Pecans
2 tbsp Light Brown Sugar
2 tbsp Granulated
1 tsp ground cinnamon
2 tbsp Whipped Butter

NUTRITION FACTS

Serving Size 1 stuffed apples

Amount per Serving

Calories 225	Calories from Fat 65.8

	% Daily Value *
Total Fat 7.31g	11%
Saturated Fat 2g	9%
Cholesterol 7.5mg	2%
Sodium 29.94mg	1%
Total Carbohydrate 44.84g	14%
Dietary Fiber 6.39g	25%
Sugars 31.38g	
Protein 1.47g	2%

Directions:
Cut off very top of apples (just enough to get stem off) and peel just around the top. Scoop out center of apples, leaving a cavity about 1 1/2 inch wide and about 1/2 inch from bottom of apple (deep). Brush peeled edges with lemon juice. Mix apricots, nuts, sugar, cinnamon, and (melted) butter well in bowl. Evenly pack each apple with mixture.
Pour 1/2 cup of water in slow cooker. Put 2 stuffed apples in bottom of slow cooker, and remaining 2 apples above but not directly on top of apples on bottom (do not cover stuffed portion with apples on top).
Cover and cook on low 3-4 hours until apples are tender. Best served warm.

<u>RESOURCES</u>

Christie, Catherine, "Mood Food Relationships," (2013) http://www.faqs.org/nutrition/Met-Obe/Mood-Food-Relationships.html

Eat Balanced (2013), www.eatbalanced.com

EZine Articles (2013), www.EzineArticles.com/4723776

Livestrong.com Demand Media (2013), Health & Wellness Site, www.livestrong.com

McKinley Health Center of the University of Illinois at Urbana-Champaign (2013), http://www.mckinley.illinois.edu/

United States Department of Agriculture (2013), http://fnic.nal.usda.gov

Wilson, Jessie (2013), www.rawfoodexplained.com